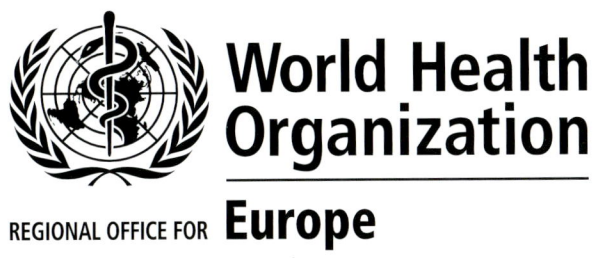
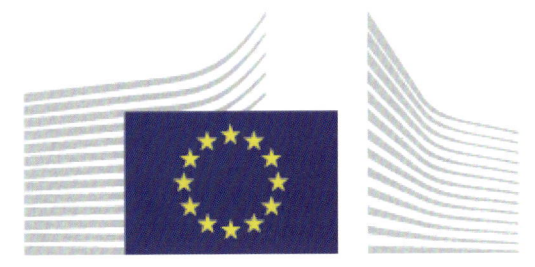

Alcohol in the European Union

Consumption, harm and policy approaches

Edited by:
Peter Anderson, Lars Møller and Gauden Galea

ABSTRACT

Alcohol is one of the world's top three priority areas in public health. Even though only half the global population drinks alcohol, it is the world's third leading cause of ill health and premature death, after low birth weight and unsafe sex, and greater than tobacco. In Europe, alcohol is also the third leading risk factor for disease and mortality after tobacco and high blood pressure. This report presents the latest literature overview of effective alcohol policies, and includes data from the European Union, Norway and Switzerland in the areas of alcohol consumption, harm and policy approaches. The data presented were collected from a survey in 2011.

Keywords

ALCOHOL DRINKING – adverse effects
ALCOHOL-RELATED DISORDERS – prevention and control
ALCOHOLISM – prevention and control
DATA COLLECTION
HARM REDUCTION
HEALTH POLICY

ISBN 978 92 890 0264 6

Address requests about publications of the WHO Regional Office for Europe to:
    Publications
    WHO Regional Office for Europe
    Scherfigsvej 8
    DK–2100 Copenhagen Ø, Denmark
Alternatively, complete an online request form for documentation, health information, or for permission to quote or translate, on the Regional Office web site (http://www.euro.who.int/pubrequest).

© World Health Organization 2012

All rights reserved. The Regional Office for Europe of the World Health Organization welcomes requests for permission to reproduce or translate its publications, in part or in full.

The designations employed and the presentation of the material in this publication do not imply the expression of any opinion whatsoever on the part of the World Health Organization concerning the legal status of any country, territory, city or area or of its authorities, or concerning the delimitation of its frontiers or boundaries. Dotted lines on maps represent approximate border lines for which there may not yet be full agreement.

The mention of specific companies or of certain manufacturers' products does not imply that they are endorsed or recommended by the World Health Organization in preference to others of a similar nature that are not mentioned. Errors and omissions excepted, the names of proprietary products are distinguished by initial capital letters.

All reasonable precautions have been taken by the World Health Organization to verify the information contained in this publication. However, the published material is being distributed without warranty of any kind, either express or implied. The responsibility for the interpretation and use of the material lies with the reader. In no event shall the World Health Organization be liable for damages arising from its use. The views expressed by authors, editors, or expert groups do not necessarily represent the decisions or the stated policy of the World Health Organization.

The responsibility for the content of this report lies with the authors and the content does not represent the views of the European Commission, nor is the Commission responsible for any use that may be made of the information contained herein.

CONTENTS

Page

Acknowledgements vi

About the authors vii

Foreword ix

Introduction 1
    Alcohol as a health issue 1
    Policy responses 2
    References 3

The impact of alcohol on health 5
    Introduction 5
    Alcohol as a carcinogen 5
    Cardiovascular disease 6
    Death 6
    Social circumstances 8
    Conclusions for policy and practice 8
    References 8

Societal burden of alcohol 10
    Introduction 10
    Alcohol consumption in Europe 10
    Alcohol-attributable burden of disease in Europe 16
    Conclusions 26
    References 26

Unrecorded and illicit alcohol 29
    Introduction 29
    Updated evidence 30
    Influence of price policies on the informal market 32
    Conclusions for practice and policy 32
    Research gaps 32
    Conclusions 33
    References 33

Information and education 35
    Introduction 35
    School-based information and education 35
    Public education campaigns 36
    Campaigns based on drinking guidelines 36
    Social responsibility messages 37
    Consumer labelling and warning messages 37
    What to do about education and information 37
    Conclusions 38
    References 38

Health sector responses 40

Introduction 40
Recent evidence 41
Conclusions for policy and practice 44
References 45

Reducing injuries and death from alcohol-related road crashes.. 49

Introduction 49
Summary of current evidence 49
Deaths and injuries from road traffic crashes with alcohol a risk factor 50
Conclusions for policy and practice 51
References 53

Community action 55

Preventive intervention at the community level... 55
Conclusions 59
References 60

Drinking environments.. 63

Introduction 63
Summary of recent evidence.. 64
Conclusions for policy and practice 66
References 66

Alcohol and the workplace 69

Introduction 69
Alcohol and employment 69
Conclusions for policy and practice 77
References 78

Availability of alcohol 83

Introduction 83
Ratings of measures controlling physical availability of alcohol 85
Conclusions for policy and practice 87
References 87

The impact of alcohol marketing.. 89

Introduction 89
Immediate effects.. 92
Conclusions for policy and practice 92
References 94

Pricing of alcohol... 96

Introduction 96
Summary of recent evidence.. 97
Affordability.. 98
Minimum prices 99
Symmetry of price elasticities.. 100
Conclusions for policy and practice 100
References 101

Overview of effectiveness and cost–effectiveness 103

    Introduction 103
    Summary of recent evidence 104
    Avoidable-burden analyses 108
    Conclusions for policy and practice 109
    References 110

Common evidence base and monitoring 111

    Introduction 111
    Monitoring approaches and their limitations 111
    European resources for monitoring 112
    Conclusions for policy and practice 115
    References 116

EU status report on public health policies on alcohol 2011 118

    Introduction 118
    Policy development at national level 118
    Price and tax measures 120
    Availability of alcoholic beverages 121
    Policies on the marketing of alcoholic beverages 124
    Information and education 126
    Community action 127
    Health sector responses 128
    Alcohol and the workplace 128
    Alcohol-free environments 129
    Drink–driving countermeasures 129
    References 132

Conclusions 133

    References 137

Annex 1 Adult per capita alcohol consumption in the EU, candidate
            countries, Norway and Switzerland (2009) 138

Annex 2 Lifetime abstainers in the EU, candidate countries,
            Norway and Switzerland by country and gender (2009) 139

Annex 3 Rates of heavy episodic drinking (binge-drinking) 140

Annex 4 Core findings and conclusions for EU-financed
            and co-financed projects since 2006 142

Acknowledgements

The WHO Regional Office for Europe is grateful to the European Commission for financial support for the production of this report.

The document was edited by Dr Peter Anderson, Consultant in Public Health, Dr Lars Møller, Programme Manager ad interim, Alcohol and Illicit Drugs and Dr Gauden Galea, Director, Noncommunicable Diseases and Health Promotion, WHO Regional Office for Europe.

WHO would like to thank all the authors for contributing to this report and Dr Ann Hope and Dr Robin Room for reviewing the document and for their valuable comments.

The document was edited for language and style by Rosemary Bohr.

About the authors

Peter Anderson MD MPH PhD FRCP
Professor, Substance Use, Policy and Practice, Institute of Health and Society, Newcastle University, United Kingdom
Professor, Alcohol and Health, Faculty of Health, Medicine and Life Sciences, Maastricht University, Netherlands

Lars Møller MD DrMSc FFPH
Programme Manager ad interim, Alcohol and Illicit Drugs, WHO Regional Office for Europe

Gauden Galea MD
Director, Division of Noncommunicable Diseases and Health Promotion, WHO Regional Office for Europe

Kevin D Shield MHSc
Centre for Addiction and Mental Health, Toronto, Canada. Institute of Medical Science, University of Toronto, Canada

Tara AK Kehoe-Chan MSc
Centre for Addiction and Mental Health, Toronto, Canada. Department of Statistics, University of Toronto, Canada

Gerrit Gmel MSc
Centre for Addiction and Mental Health, Toronto, Canada

Maximilien X Rehm
Faculty of Arts and Sciences/Politics and Governance, Ryerson University, Toronto, Canada

Jürgen Rehm PhD
Director, Social and Epidemiological Research Department, Centre for Addiction and Mental Health, Toronto, Canada
Senior Scientist and Head, Population Health Research Group, Centre for Addiction and Mental Health, Canada
Professor and Chairperson, Addiction Policy, Dalla Lana School of Public Health, University of Toronto, Canada
Professor, Department of Psychiatry, Faculty of Medicine, University of Toronto, Canada
Head, PAHO/WHO Collaborating Centre for Mental Health & Addiction
Head, Epidemiological Research Unit, Technische Universität Dresden, Klinische Psychologie & Psychotherapie, Dresden, Germany
Faculty member: Graduate Department of Community Health and Institute of Medical Science, University of Toronto, Canada

Dirk Lachenmeier PhD
Head, Alcohol Laboratory, Chemical and Veterinary Investigation Agency, Karlsruhe, Germany

Eileen Kaner PhD
Institute Director and Professor of Public Health Research, Institute of Health and Society, Newcastle University, United Kingdom

Francesco Mitis
Violence and Injury Prevention, WHO Regional Office for Europe

Dinesh Sethi MSc MD MRCP FFPH
Programme Manager ad interim, Violence and Injury Prevention, WHO Regional Office for Europe

Allaman Allamani MD
Agenzia Regionale di Sanità, Regione Toscana, Firenze, Italy

Karen Hughes PhD
Reader, Centre for Public Health, Liverpool John Moores University, United Kingdom

Mark Bellis PhD DSc FFPH
Professor, Centre for Public Health, Liverpool John Moores University, United Kingdom

Esa Österberg MSc
Senior Researcher, Department of Alcohol, Drugs and Addiction, National Institute for Health and Welfare, Helsinki, Finland

Avalon de Bruijn MSc
Coordinator, Alcohol Marketing Europe, European Centre for Monitoring Alcohol Marketing, Utrecht, Netherlands

Jacek Moskalewicz PhD
Head, Department of Studies on Alcoholism and Drug Dependence, Institute of Psychiatry and Neurology, Warsaw, Poland

Julie Brummer MPH
Consultant, WHO Regional Office for Europe

Lis Sevestre MPH
Consultant, WHO Regional Office for Europe

Foreword

In 2008, the European Commission and the WHO Regional Office for Europe started a project to establish a European Information System on Alcohol and Health, to replace the alcohol information system dating from 2002. This work was carried out in close collaboration with the Department of Mental Health and Substance Abuse at WHO headquarters in Geneva as part of the Global Information System on Alcohol and Health. As a result, the European status report on alcohol and health *was produced in 2010, based on information gathered in 2009 across the WHO European Region. This new report on alcohol in the European Union uses information gathered in 2011 to update key indicators on alcohol consumption, health outcomes and action to reduce harm across the European Union (EU).*

Cooperation between WHO and the European Commission on data-gathering and analysis underpins the development of effective public health policies to reduce alcohol-related harm in the EU and in the wider WHO European Region.

The European Region was the first of the WHO regions to adopt an Alcohol Action Plan, in 1992. In May 2010, the Sixty-third World Health Assembly adopted the Global Strategy to Reduce the Harmful Use of Alcohol. At the Sixty-First session of the WHO Regional Committee for Europe in September 2011, Member States adopted the European Action Plan to Reduce the Harmful Use of Alcohol 2012–2020.

In 2006, the EU strategy to support member states in reducing alcohol-related harm was launched. This strategy focuses on: (i) protecting young people, children and the unborn child; (ii) reducing injuries and death from alcohol-related road accidents; (iii) preventing alcohol-related harm among adults and reducing the negative impact on the workplace; (iv) informing, educating and raising awareness about the impact of harmful and hazardous alcohol consumption and about appropriate consumption patterns; and (v) developing and maintaining a common evidence base at EU level.

As highlighted in the EU strategy, research and information systems are crucial for the development and implementation of effective action at EU, national and local level. The Global Strategy to Reduce the Harmful Use of Alcohol stresses similarly that local, national and international monitoring and surveillance are needed in order to monitor the magnitude of and trends in alcohol-related harm, to strengthen advocacy, to formulate policies and to assess the impact of interventions.

Since the 1970s, the WHO Regional Office has promoted an evidence-based approach to alcohol policies, including through a series of publications to summarize current knowledge of the effectiveness and cost–effectiveness of various policy approaches. In 2006, a comprehensive compilation of research-based knowledge on public health aspects of alcohol was prepared by the Institute of Alcohol Studies for the European Commission, to inform the preparation of the EU strategy to support member states in reducing alcohol-related harm.

This report on alcohol in the European Union updates the evidence base for some important areas of alcohol policy, drawing in particular on literature published since the launch of the EU strategy. It is noteworthy that the most recent evidence confirms and expands previous knowledge and does not alter fundamental findings and conclusions.

Zsuzsanna Jakab
WHO Regional Director for Europe

Introduction

Lars Møller and Peter Anderson

Alcohol as a health issue

Alcohol is one of the world's top three priority public health areas. Even though only half the global population drinks alcohol, it is the world's third leading cause of ill health and premature death, after low birth weight and unsafe sex (for which alcohol is a risk factor), and greater than tobacco. In Europe, alcohol is also the third leading risk factor for disease and mortality after tobacco and high blood pressure (WHO, 2009).

The European Union (EU) is the region with the highest alcohol consumption in the world: in 2009, average adult (aged 15+ years) alcohol consumption in the EU was 12.5 litres of pure alcohol – 27g of pure alcohol or nearly three drinks a day, more than double the world average. Although there are many individual country differences, alcohol consumption in the EU as a whole has continued at a stable level over the past decade. Alcohol is a cause of noncommunicable diseases, including cancers, cardiovascular diseases and liver diseases; communicable diseases, increasing the risks of HIV/AIDS, tuberculosis and community-acquired pneumonia; and all types of intentional and unintentional injury, including homicides and suicides. Alcohol harms people other than the drinker, whether through violence on the street, domestic violence in the family, or simply using government resources, notably through the costs of providing health care, unemployment and incapacity benefits, and dealing with crime and disorder.

The harms from drinking disproportionately affect poorer people. Socially disadvantaged people and people who live in socially disadvantaged areas experience more harm from the same dose of alcohol than those who are better off. Increased spending on social welfare policies can mitigate the impact of economic downturns and unemployment on increased alcohol-related deaths.

The real absolute risk of dying from an adverse alcohol-related condition increases with the total amount of alcohol consumed over a lifetime. Most alcohol is drunk in heavy drinking occasions, which worsen all risks, including ischaemic heart disease and sudden death.

Alcohol can diminish individual health and human capital throughout the lifespan from the embryo to old age. In absolute terms, it is mostly middle-aged people (men in particular) who die from alcohol. Taking into account a life-course view, however, exposure to alcohol during pregnancy can impair the brain development of the fetus and is associated with intellectual deficits that become apparent later in childhood. The adolescent brain is particularly susceptible to alcohol, and the longer the onset of consumption is delayed, the less likely it is that alcohol-related problems and alcohol dependence will emerge in adult life. In the workplace, harmful alcohol use and heavy episodic drinking increase the risk of problems such as absenteeism, presenteeism (low productivity) and inappropriate behaviour. Workplaces, themselves, can also increase the risk of alcohol use disorders and alcohol dependence.

Policy responses

The WHO Regional Office for Europe has a long history of taking action on alcohol. It was the first regional office to address the problem, starting in 1975 with the scientific publication *Alcohol control policies in a public health perspective* (Bruun et al., 1975). This was followed by two further scientific publications, *Alcohol policy and the public good* by Edwards et al. (1994) and *Alcohol, no ordinary commodity* by Babor et al. (2003; 2010). At a political level, action culminated in the *European Alcohol Action Plan 1992–1999*, first endorsed by the Member States in 1992, which was complemented by the *European Charter on Alcohol* in 1995 and updated in 2000 (WHO Regional Office for Europe, 1992; 1995; 2000). In 2006, the Member States endorsed the *Framework for alcohol policy in the WHO European Region*, which provides a frame for implementing the European Alcohol Action Plan (WHO Regional Office for Europe, 2006), and in September 2011 a new *European Action Plan to Reduce the Harmful Use of Alcohol 2012–2020* was adopted by the Regional Committee (WHO Regional Office for Europe, 2011). More recent publications include the *European status report on alcohol and health 2010, Evidence for the effectiveness and cost–effectiveness of interventions to reduce alcohol-related harm* and *Handbook for action to reduce alcohol-related harm* (WHO Regional Office for Europe, 2009a; 2009b; 2010). The work of the Region was given a boost in 2010 with the adoption of the WHO *Global strategy to reduce the harmful use of alcohol* (WHO, 2010).

In the EU, strategy-level work on alcohol and health took longer to start. Although the internal market framework has affected alcohol policy issues throughout the history of the European Community and the EU (Sulkunen, 1982), specific action on alcohol as a public health issue can be said to have started in 2001, with European Council conclusions inviting the European Commission (EC) to develop a Community strategy to reduce alcohol-related harm (European Council, 2001a) and a Council recommendation to address drinking by young people, particularly children and adolescents (European Council, 2001b). At about the same time, the European Parliament and Council adopted a programme of Community action in the field of public health (2003–2008) with financing available for alcohol projects, a provision that was later renewed in a second programme (2008–2013) (European Council, 2002; 2007). EU action on alcohol culminated in 2006 with a Commission Communication on an EU strategy to support member states in reducing alcohol-related harm (European Commission, 2006). The Communication highlighted five priority themes: protecting young people, children and the unborn child; reducing injuries and death from alcohol-related road accidents; preventing alcohol-related harm among adults and reducing the negative impact on the workplace; informing, educating and raising awareness about the impact of harmful and hazardous alcohol consumption, and about appropriate consumption patterns; and developing and maintaining a common evidence base at EU level.

The first two chapters of this report highlight the harm that alcohol can do to individuals, societies and communities. These are followed by a third chapter which, while reminding of the potential harm from illicit alcohol, concludes that this is probably not a major health problem for the EU. There then follows a series of chapters summarizing and reporting on new evidence of effectiveness of various public health policies on alcohol, published since a comprehensive compilation of research-based knowledge on public health aspects of alcohol (Anderson & Baumberg, 2006) was prepared for the European Commission to inform the preparation of the EU strategy. The fields covered are: information and education, health sector responses, reduction of injuries and deaths from alcohol-related road crashes, community action, drinking environments, alcohol and the workplace, the availability of alcohol, the marketing of alcohol and the price of alcohol. Where appropriate, each chapter also summarizes some of the key alcohol-related projects and activities that have been financed or co-financed by the Commission. The nine policy-focused chapters are followed by a chapter summarizing what is known about the cost–effectiveness of implementing different polices, and then a chapter on a common evidence base and monitoring. The chapter on the EU status report on alcohol consumption, health outcomes and policies represents the results of a survey carried out in 2011, reporting the situation as at 31 December 2010. The chapter notes that while there is still a long way to go and policy has yet to result in noticeable impacts in reductions of per capita alcohol consumption (the main determinant of harm), the implementation of alcohol policies has clearly moved forward over the past five or six years. A final chapter of conclusions brings everything together and stresses the importance of implementing evidence-based policy to improve the health and well-being of European citizens as well as supporting the sustainability and productivity of the EU as a whole.

References

Anderson P, Baumberg B (2006). *Alcohol in Europe. A public health perspective.* London, Institute of Alcohol Studies (http://ec.europa.eu/health-eu/doc/alcoholineu_content_en.pdf, accessed 18 February 2012).

Babor TF et al. (2003). *Alcohol: no ordinary commodity. Research and public policy.* Oxford, Oxford University Press.

Babor TF et al. (2010). *Alcohol: no ordinary commodity*, 2nd ed. Oxford, Oxford University Press.

Bruun K et al. (1975). *Alcohol control policies in public health perspective.* Helsinki, Finnish Foundation for Alcohol Studies.

Edwards G et al. (1994). *Alcohol policy and the public good.* New York, Oxford University Press.

European Commission (2006). *Communication from the Commission to the Council, the European Parliament, the European Economic and Social Committee and the Committee of the Regions. An EU strategy to support Member States in reducing alcohol related harm.* Brussels, Commission of the European Communities (COM(2006) 625 final) (http://eur-lex.europa.eu/LexUriServ/site/en/com/2006/com2006_0625en01.pdf, accessed 21 February 2012).

European Council (2001a). Council conclusions of 5 June 2001 on a Community strategy to reduce alcohol-related harm (2001/C 175/01). *Official Journal of the European Communities,* 44(C 175):1–2 (http://eur-lex.europa.eu/LexUriServ/LexUriServ.do?uri=OJ:C:2001:175:0001:0002:en:pdf, accessed 7 February 2012).

European Council (2001b). Council recommendation of 5 June 2001 on the drinking of alcohol by young people, in particular children and adolescents (2001/458/EC). *Official Journal of the European Communities,* 44(L 161):38–41 (http://eur-lex.europa.eu/LexUriServ/LexUriServ.do?uri=OJ:L:2001:161:0038:0041:EN:PDF, accessed 7 February 2012).

European Council (2002). Decision No. 1786/2002/EC of the European Parliament and of the Council of 23 September 2002 adopting a programme of Community action in the field of public health (2003–2008). *Official Journal of the European Communities*, 45(L 271):1–11 (http://eur-lex.europa.eu/LexUriServ/LexUri Serv.do?uri=OJ:L:2002:271:0001:0011:EN:PDF, accessed 7 February 2012).

European Council (2007). Decision No. 1350/2007/EC of the European Parliament and of the Council of 23 October 2007 establishing a second programme of Community action in the field of health (2008–13). *Official Journal of the European Communities*, 50(L 301):3–13 (http://eur-lex.europa.eu/LexUriServ/LexUriServ.do?uri=OJ:L:2007:301:0003:0013:EN:PDF, accessed 7 February 2012).

Sulkunen P (1982). Economic integration and the availability of alcohol: the case of the European Economic Community. *Contemporary Drug Problems*, 10(1):75–102.

WHO (2009). *Global health risks*. Geneva, World Health Organization (http://www.who.int/healthinfo/global_burden_disease/global_health_risks/en/index.html, accessed 7 February 2012).

WHO (2010). *Global strategy to reduce the harmful use of alcohol*. Geneva, World Health Organization (http://www.who.int/substance_abuse/msbalcstragegy.pdf, accessed 18 February 2012).

WHO Regional Office for Europe (1992). *European Alcohol Action Plan 1992–1999*. Copenhagen, WHO Regional Office for Europe.

WHO Regional Office for Europe (1995). *European Charter on Alcohol adopted at the European Conference on Health, Society and Alcohol, Paris, 12–14 December 1995*. Copenhagen, WHO Regional Office for Europe (http://www.euro.who.int/__data/assets/pdf_file/0008/79406/EUR_ICP_ALDT_94_03_CN01.pdf, accessed 7 February 2012).

WHO Regional Office for Europe (2000). *European Alcohol Action Plan 2000–2005*. Copenhagen, WHO Regional Office for Europe (http://www.euro.who.int/document/E67946.pdf, accessed 7 February 2012).

WHO Regional Office for Europe (2006). *Framework for alcohol policy in the WHO European Region*. Copenhagen, WHO Regional Office for Europe (http://www.euro.who.int/document/e88335.pdf, accessed 7 February 2012).

WHO Regional Office for Europe (2009a). *Evidence for the effectiveness and cost–effectiveness of interventions to reduce alcohol-related harm*. Copenhagen, WHO Regional Office for Europe (http://www.euro.who.int/__data/assets/pdf_file/0020/43319/E92823.pdf, accessed 12 February 2012).

WHO Regional Office for Europe (2009b). *Handbook for action to reduce alcohol-related harm*. Copenhagen, WHO Regional Office for Europe (http://www.euro.who.int/__data/assets/pdf_file/0012/43320/E92820.pdf, accessed 7 February 2012).

WHO Regional Office for Europe (2010). *European status report on alcohol and health 2010*. Copenhagen, WHO Regional Office for Europe (http://www.euro.who.int/__data/assets/pdf_file/0004/128065/e94533.pdf, accessed 7 February 2012).

WHO Regional Office for Europe (2011). *European Action Plan to Reduce the Harmful Use of Alcohol 2012–2020*. Copenhagen, WHO Regional Office for Europe (EUR/RC61/13, + EUR/RC61/Conf.Doc./6; (http://www.euro.who.int/__data/assets/pdf_file/0006/147732/wd13E_Alcohol_111372.pdf, accessed 7 February 2012).

The impact of alcohol on health

Peter Anderson

Introduction

Apart from being a drug of dependence, alcohol has been known for many years as a cause of some 60 different types of disease and condition, including injuries, mental and behavioural disorders, gastrointestinal conditions, cancers, cardiovascular diseases, immunological disorders, lung diseases, skeletal and muscular diseases, reproductive disorders and pre-natal harm, including an increased risk of prematurity and low birth weight (Anderson & Baumberg, 2006). In recent years, overwhelming evidence has confirmed that both the volume of lifetime alcohol use and the combination of frequency of drinking and amount drunk per incident increase the risk of alcohol-related harm, largely in a dose-dependent manner (WHO Regional Office for Europe, 2009; Rehm et al., 2010) with the higher the alcohol consumption, the greater the risk. For some conditions, such as cardiomyopathy, acute respiratory distress syndrome and muscle damage, harm appears only to result from a sustained level of high alcohol consumption, but even at high levels, alcohol increases the risk and severity of these conditions in a dose-dependent manner. The frequency and volume of episodic heavy drinking are of particular importance for increasing the risk of injuries and certain cardiovascular diseases (coronary heart disease and stroke). Although there is a protective effect of light to moderate drinking on ischaemic diseases, overwhelmingly alcohol is toxic to the cardiovascular system.

Alcohol is an intoxicant affecting a wide range of structures and processes in the central nervous system which, interacting with personality characteristics, associated behaviour and sociocultural expectations, are causal factors for intentional and unintentional injuries and harm to both the drinker and others. These injuries and harm include interpersonal violence, suicide, homicide and drink–driving fatalities. Alcohol consumption is a risk factor for risky sexual behaviour, sexually transmitted diseases and HIV infection. Moreover, it is a potent teratogen with a range of negative outcomes to the fetus, including low birth weight, cognitive deficiencies and fetal alcohol disorders. It is neurotoxic to brain development, leading to structural changes in the hippocampus in adolescence and reduced brain volume in middle age. Alcohol is a dependence-producing drug, similar to other substances under international control. The process of dependence occurs through its reinforcing properties and neuroadaptation. It is also an immunosuppressant which increases the risk of communicable diseases, including tuberculosis. Further, alcoholic beverages and the ethanol in them are classified as carcinogens by the International Agency for Research on Cancer.

Alcohol as a carcinogen

In 2007, the International Agency for Research on Cancer concluded that there was a causal link between alcohol and cancer of the oral cavity, pharynx, larynx, oesophagus, liver, colon, rectum and female breast (Baan et al., 2007; IARC, 2010). All these cancers showed evidence of a dose–response relationship; that is, the risk of cancer increases steadily with greater volumes of drinking (Rehm et al., 2010). The strength of the relationship to levels of average alcohol consumption varies for different cancers. For example, with regard to female breast cancer, each additional 10 g of pure alcohol per day is associated with an increase of 7% in the relative risk of breast cancer, whereas regular consumption of approximately 50 g of pure alcohol increases the relative risk of colorectal cancer by 10–20%, indicating that the association is stronger for female breast cancer. Conversely, the relationship of average consumption to cancer of the larynx, pharynx and oesophagus is markedly higher than the relationship to both breast and colorectal cancer (more than a 100% increase for an average consumption of 50 g pure alcohol per day). Among the causal mechanisms that have been indicated for some cancers is the toxic effect of acetaldehyde, which is a metabolite of alcohol.

Cardiovascular disease

Alcohol use is related overwhelmingly detrimentally to many cardiovascular outcomes, including hypertensive disease (Taylor et al., 2009), haemorrhagic stroke (Patra et al., 2010) and atrial fibrillation (Samokhvalov, Irving & Rehm, 2010). For ischaemic heart disease and ischaemic stroke, the relationship is more complex. Chronic heavy alcohol use has been associated uniformly with adverse cardiovascular outcomes (Rehm & Roerecke, 2011). But, on average, light to moderate drinking has a protective effect on ischaemic diseases (Roerecke & Rehm, in press). This effect is found to be equal for people who just drink beer or who just drink wine (Di Castelnuovo et al., 2002). More and more, however, it is being understood that a large part of this effect is due to confounders (Roerecke & Rehm, 2010), with low to moderate alcohol use being a proxy for better health and social capital (Hansel et al., 2010). In any case, the protective effect totally disappears when drinkers report at least one heavy drinking occasion per month (Roerecke & Rehm, 2010); there is no protective effect for younger people, for whom any dose of alcohol increases the risk of ischaemic events (Juonala et al., 2009); and, in older people, a greater reduction in death from ischaemic heart disease can be more effectively obtained by being physically active and eating a healthier diet than by drinking a low dose of alcohol (Mukamal et al., 2006). The detrimental effects of heavy drinking occasions on ischaemic diseases are consistent with the physiological mechanisms of increased clotting and a reduced threshold for ventricular fibrillation which occur following heavy drinking (Rehm et al., 2010).

Death

It is mostly the middle-aged (and men in particular) who die from alcohol (Jones et al., 2009; Rehm, Zatonski & Taylor, 2011). Taking into account a lifecourse view, however, the adolescent brain is particularly susceptible to alcohol, and the longer the onset of consumption is delayed, the less likely that alcohol-related problems and alcohol dependence will emerge in adult life (Norberg, Bierut & Grucza, 2009). The absolute real risk of dying from an adverse alcohol-related condition increases linearly with the amount of alcohol consumed over a lifetime, with no safe level (Rehm, Zatonski & Taylor, 2011). In many societies there is no difference in the risks between men and women. Australians who regularly drink six drinks (60 g of alcohol) a day over their lives as adults have a 1 in 10 chance of dying from alcohol (National Health and Medical Research Council, 2009).

The annual absolute risk of dying from an alcohol-related disease (accounting for the protective effect of ischaemic diseases) for people aged over 15 years across the population of the WHO European Region is shown in Fig. 1. The risks increase from the consumption of 10 g alcohol a day (one drink, the lowest data point) so that at a consumption of 60 g/day, men have a just under 9% annual risk of dying from an alcohol-related disease and women an 8% risk. At any given level of alcohol consumption, men are at greater risk than women. The lifetime risk of dying from an alcohol-related injury across the total population aged over 15 years rises exponentially with an increasing daily alcohol consumption beyond 10 g of alcohol per day, the first data point (Fig. 2). At any given level of alcohol consumption, the risks are much higher for men than for women.

Fig. 1. Absolute annual risk of death from alcohol-related diseases[a]

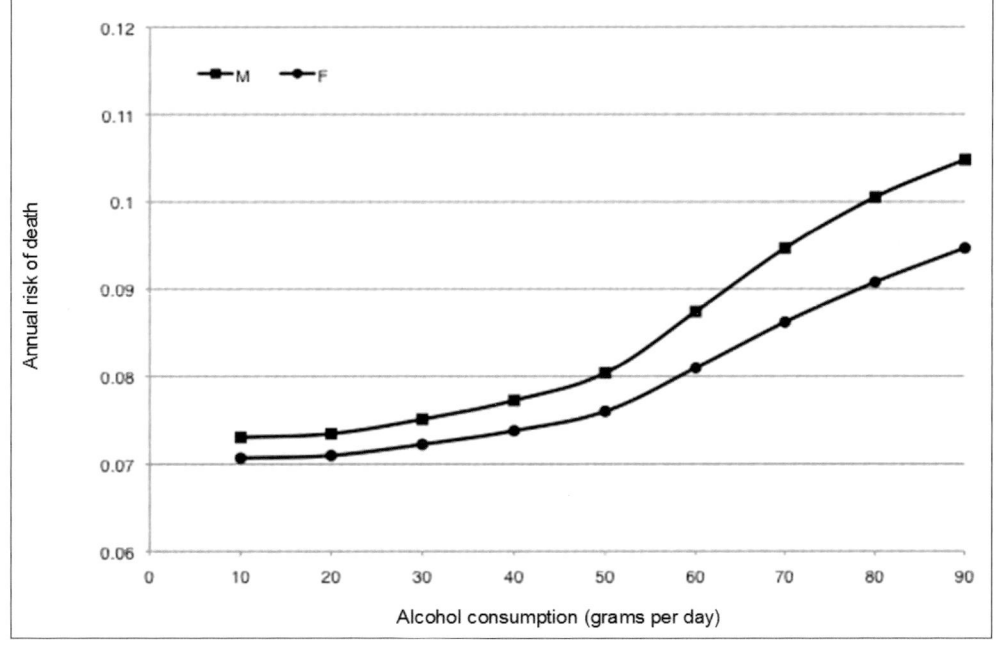

[a] Absolute annual risk of death from alcohol dependence, liver cirrhosis and alcohol-related cancers and cardiovascular diseases, net of protective effects, from drinking a certain average amount of alcohol daily from 10 g alcohol/day to 90 g/day, age-standardized for adults aged over 15 years for the WHO European Region (*Source:* Taylor, Rehm & Anderson, 2010, personal information).

Fig. 2. Life-time risk of death from alcohol-related injuries[a]

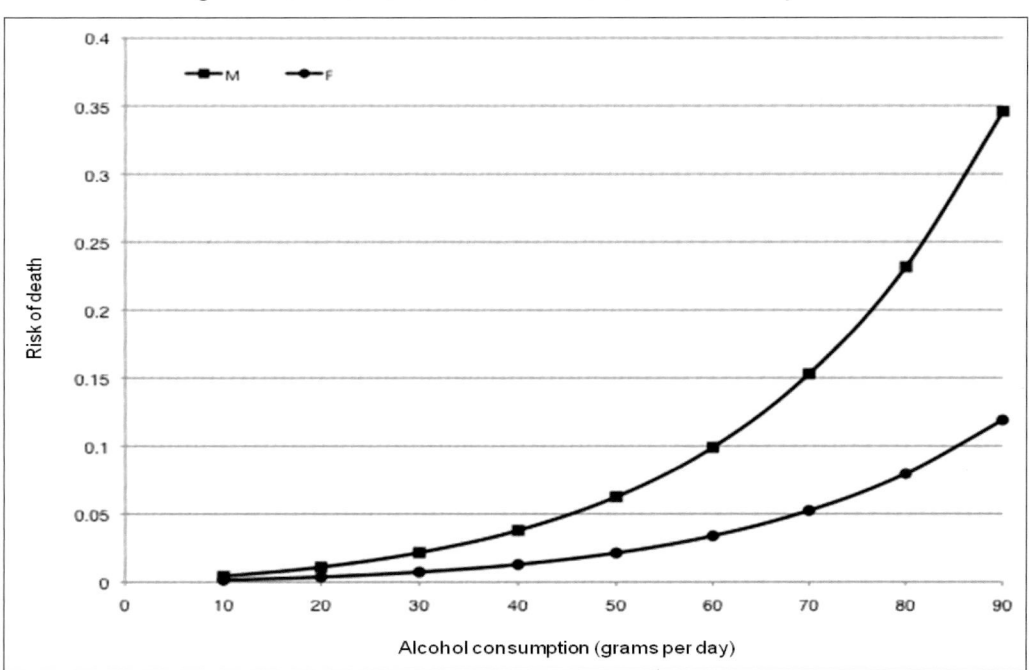

[a] Absolute lifetime risk of death from alcohol-related intentional and unintentional injuries from drinking a certain average amount of alcohol daily from 10 g alcohol/day to 90 g/day, age-standardized for adults aged over 15 years for the WHO European Region (*Source:* Taylor, Rehm & Anderson, 2010, personal information).

Social circumstances

People who are socially disadvantaged people or who live in socially disadvantaged areas experience more harm per gram of alcohol consumed than the better-off (Rehm et al., 2009). In Finland, areas with higher levels of manual workers or of unemployment and areas with lower social cohesion had higher levels of alcohol-related mortality among men aged 25–64 years (Blomgren, Martikainen & Makela, 2004). In the same way, social networks matter. Changes in alcohol consumption among a person's social network have a significant effect on that person's subsequent behaviour, in terms of not drinking (when more of the network abstain) or of drinking heavily (when more of the network drink heavily) (Rosenquist, Murabito & Fowler, 2010).

Conclusions for policy and practice

The following conclusions should be helpful for policy and practice.

- The risk of death from an alcohol-related illness or injury rises with increasing alcohol consumption.

- At 20 g of alcohol consumed on average per day or per drinking occasion per day (at least for the Australian population), the lifetime risk of death from an acute or chronic condition is less than 1 in 100.

- For a given level of alcohol consumption, people from lower socioeconomic groups are at increased risk of an alcohol-related death, compounded by living in areas with a higher degree of disadvantage.

- Incentives need to be implemented (Anderson et al., 2011) that make it easier for individuals to drink less alcohol per day and per occasion (Anderson, Harrison & Cooper, 2011).

References

Anderson P, Baumberg B (2006). *Alcohol in Europe. A public health perspective*. London, Institute of Alcohol Studies (http://ec.europa.eu/health-eu/doc/alcoholineu_content_en.pdf, accessed 18 February 2012).

Anderson P et al. (2011). Communicating alcohol narratives: creating a healthier relation with alcohol. *Journal of Health Communication*, 16(S2):27–36.

Anderson P, Harrison O, Cooper C (2011). Incentives for health. *Journal of Health Communication*, 16(S2):107–133.

Baan R et al. (2007). Carcinogenicity of alcoholic beverages. *The Lancet Oncology*, 8:292–293.

Blomgren J, Martikainen P, Makela P (2004). The effects of regional characteristics on alcohol-related mortality – a register-based multilevel analysis of 1.1 million men. *Social Science & Medicine*, 58:2523–2535.

Di Castelnuovo A et al. (2002). Meta-analysis of wine and beer consumption in relation to vascular risk. *Circulation*, 105(24):2836–2844.

Hansel B et al. (2010). Relationship between alcohol intake, health and social status and cardiovascular risk factors in the urban Paris-Ile-De-France cohort: is the cardioprotective action of alcohol a myth? *European Journal of Clinical Nutrition*, 64:561–568.

International Agency for Research on Cancer (2010). *Alcohol consumption and ethyl carbamate*. Lyons, International Agency for Research on Cancer.

Jones L et al. (2009). *Alcohol-attributable fraction for England. Alcohol-attributable mortality and hospital admissions*. Liverpool John Moores University, Centre for Public Health, Northwest Public Health Observatory (http://www.nwph.net/nwpho/Publications/Alcohol AttributableFractions.pdf, accessed 14 February 2012).

Juonala M et al. (2009). Alcohol consumption is directly associated with carotid intima-media thickness in Finnish young adults. The Cardiovascular Risk in Young Finns study. *Atherosclerosis*, 204:e93–e98.

Mukamal K et al. (2006). Alcohol consumption and the risk of coronary heart disease in older adults: the Cardiovascular Health Study. *Journal of the American Geriatric Society*, 54:30–37.

National Health and Medical Research Council (2009). *Australian guidelines to reduce health risks from drinking alcohol*. Canberra, National Health and Medical Research Council.

Norberg KE, Bierut LJ, Grucza RA (2009). Long-term effects of minimum drinking age laws on past-year alcohol and drug use disorders. *Alcoholism: Clinical and Experimental Research*, 33(12):2180–2190.

Patra J et al. (2010). Alcohol consumption and the risk of morbidity and mortality from different stroke types – a systematic review and meta-analysis. *BMC Public Health,* 10: 258.

Rehm J et al. (2009). *Alcohol, social development and infectious disease*. Toronto, Centre for Addiction and Mental Health.

Rehm J et al. (2010). The relation between different dimensions of alcohol consumption and burden of disease – an overview. *Addiction,* 105:817–843.

Rehm J, Roerecke M (2011). Alcohol, the heart and the cardiovascular system – what do we know and where should we go? *Drug and Alcohol Review,* 30:335–337.

Rehm J, Zatonski W, Taylor B (2011). Epidemiology and alcohol policy in Europe. *Addiction*, 106(Suppl. 1): 11–19.

Roerecke M, Rehm J (2010). Irregular heavy drinking occasions and risk of ischemic heart disease: a systematic review and meta-analysis. *American Journal of Epidemiology,* 171:633–644.

Roerecke M, Rehm J (in press). The cardioprotective association of average alcohol consumption and ischaemic heart disease: a systematic review and meta-analysis. *Addiction*.

Rosenquist JN, Murabito J, Fowler JH (2010). The spread of alcohol consumption behaviour in a large social network. *Annals of Internal Medicine,* 152:426–433.

Samokhvalov AV, Irving HM, Rehm J (2010). Alcohol as a risk factor for atrial fibrillation: a systematic review and meta-analysis. *European Journal of Cardiovascular Prevention and Rehabilitation*, 17:706–712.

Taylor B et al. (2009). Alcohol and hypertension: gender differences in dose–response relationships determined through systematic review and meta-analysis. *Addiction,* 104:1981–1990.

WHO Regional Office for Europe (2009). *Evidence for the effectiveness and cost–effectiveness of interventions to reduce alcohol-related harm*. Copenhagen, WHO Regional Office for Europe (http://www.euro.who.int/__data/assets/pdf_file/0020/43319/E92823.pdf, accessed 12 February 2012).

Societal burden of alcohol

Kevin D Shield, Tara Kehoe, Gerrit Gmel, Maximilien X Rehm and Jürgen Rehm

Introduction

Alcohol consumption has been deeply embedded in European culture for centuries, making the study of the harm it causes essential. The current volume of alcohol consumption in the EU has been stable for several years at a high level and is still more than double the global level. Patterns of drinking vary, with more irregular heavy drinking occasions in Nordic, central-eastern and eastern European countries.

Average volumes of alcohol consumption and patterns of drinking affect both health and social outcomes. In the EU in 2004, conservative estimates indicate that almost 95 000 men and over 25 000 women aged between 15 and 64 years died of alcohol-attributable causes (total 120 000, corresponding to 11.8% of all deaths in this age category). This means that 1 in 7 male deaths and 1 in 13 female deaths in this age category were caused by alcohol. These are net numbers; the protective effect of alcohol on ischaemic disease and diabetes has been taken into consideration.

Moreover, as alcohol consumption contributes substantially to morbidity and disability, the overall alcohol-attributable burden of disease is high. Partial estimates indicate that in 2004, over four million disability-adjusted life-years (DALYs) – years of life lost due to either premature mortality or to disability – were caused by alcohol consumption in the EU, corresponding to 15% of all DALYs in men and 4% of all DALYs in women (again net numbers). It is, therefore, clear that alcohol consumption is responsible for a substantial health burden within the EU.

There are additional social and economic burdens resulting from the effects of alcohol consumption on the individual, family, work and society. Many of these burdens affect people other than the drinker, and while full quantification of the harm to others is difficult, the data available for Europe suggest that there is a large impact. In the EU in 2004, over 7000 deaths and 200 000 DALYs were caused by harm to others attributable to alcohol consumption.

In theory, all alcohol-related burdens are avoidable. The remainder of this book will examine the best ways to reduce this burden.

Alcohol consumption in Europe

Patterns of drinking in different European regions

Alcohol consumption in Europe[1] has a long history spanning several thousand years (Anderson & Baumberg, 2006; McGovern, 2007), with both the Greeks and the Romans being examples of societies with a fairly widespread use of alcohol (McGovern, 2007; Phillips, 2000). Alcohol consumption is, however, differently embedded in the cultures of various countries (Iontchev, 1998; Leifman, 2002; Popova et al., 2007; Room, 2010; Room & Mäkelä, 2000). Without too much simplification, the following regional patterns can be distinguished based on the economic power of the countries, their history, average volume of consumption, drinking patterns and social reactions to alcohol.

---

[1] If not otherwise specified, Europe in this chapter will be defined as the EU plus Norway and Switzerland.

- *Central-eastern and eastern Europe.* All these countries (Bulgaria, Czech Republic, Estonia, Hungary, Latvia, Lithuania, Poland, Romania, Slovakia and Slovenia) are relatively new in the EU and have, on average, lower economic power than the rest of the EU. In 2005, their gross domestic product (GDP)-purchasing power parity (PPP) was, on average, less than half the EU average. Alcohol consumption is, on average, higher than in the rest of the EU with, in most countries, a higher rate of unrecorded consumption and a pattern of irregular heavy drinking occasions (Popova et al., 2007; Zatonski et al., 2008). Traditionally, spirits were the alcoholic beverage of choice or played a relatively large role in most of these countries (WHO, 2004), even in central European beer-drinking countries such as the Czech Republic and Slovakia, and in more wine-drinking countries such as Bulgaria, Hungary, Romania and Slovenia.

- *Central-western and western Europe* (Austria, Belgium, France, Germany, Ireland, Luxembourg, Netherlands, Switzerland, United Kingdom)[2] comprises five of the six founding members of the EU (Belgium, France, Germany, Luxembourg, Netherlands), two countries from the first enlargements (Ireland, United Kingdom) plus Austria, which joined later, and Switzerland, which is not a member of the EU but tied to it by many bilateral treaties. This region is characterized by high GDP (PPP), about 10% above the EU average. In terms of alcohol consumption, beer has been the preferred beverage in all countries with the exception of France. The drinking pattern in recent decades has overall been similar to the Mediterranean style, both in frequency of drinking and lack of acceptance of public drunkenness, with the exceptions of Ireland and the United Kingdom which are closer to the Nordic countries in this respect. It should be noted that there were times in the past of different drinking styles and much more acceptance of intoxication in Germany (Spode, 1993) or the Netherlands (Room, 1992). In addition, in central-western Europe there is more consumption between meals, and there are more alcohol-related problems compared to southern Europe.

- The pattern in the *Nordic countries* (Denmark, Finland, Iceland, Norway and Sweden) relies on drinking spirits, and is traditionally found in the northern and north-eastern parts of Europe. The use of spirits in recreational drinking spread only after 1500 and thus has a substantially shorter tradition than does wine-drinking in the Mediterranean region (see below). The traditional pattern of drinking spirits in these countries can be characterized by non-daily drinking, irregular heavy and very heavy drinking episodes (such as during weekends and at festivities) and a higher level of acceptance of drunkenness in public (Room, 2010; Room & Mäkelä, 2000). The overall volume of alcohol consumption in Nordic countries has been lower than the EU average. Even though this drinking pattern can still be observed today, spirits are no longer the dominant alcoholic beverage and there are some differences between the countries involved, with Denmark having a more central-western and western style of drinking (Mäkelä et al., 2001). This region has the highest GDP-PPP.

- The countries of *southern Europe* (Cyprus, Greece, Italy, Malta, Portugal, Spain) have a Mediterranean drinking pattern. In the south of the EU wine has traditionally been produced and drunk, characterized by almost daily drinking of alcohol (often wine with meals), avoidance of irregular heavy drinking and no acceptance of public drunkenness (Anderson & Baumberg, 2006). The overall volume of consumption has traditionally been high, except in Cyprus and Malta, but it has been falling over recent decades (WHO, 2004, 2011; see also the discussion on trends, below).

---

[2] Other classifications place France as part of southern Europe. Drinking patterns in Ireland and the United Kingdom are now closer to the Nordic countries than to the rest of this grouping.

As there are more differences in drinking patterns and environments between these regions than within them, this categorization of countries will be used throughout this chapter.

Indicators for alcohol consumption in Europe

The best indicator for overall volume of alcohol consumption is adult (age 15+ years) per capita consumption (Gmel & Rehm, 2004), as it avoids the various biases introduced by current surveys of the general population (for example, Groves, 2004; Shield & Rehm, 2012). Adult per capita consumption is usually derived from sales and taxation, but can also be derived from production and export and import figures (Rehm et al., 2003; Rehm, Klotsche & Patra, 2007). Using this indicator, adult citizens of the EU drink 12.5 litres of pure alcohol per year or 26.9 g of pure alcohol per day (this corresponds to more than 2 standard drinks of 12 g pure alcohol per day^3). In the EU, more than twice the amount of alcohol is consumed per capita than is consumed globally; the global average in 2004 was 6.1 litres adult per capita consumption (WHO, 2011).

Table 1 provides an overview of regional differences. As indicated above, alcohol consumption in Europe is highest in the central-eastern and eastern countries and lowest in the Nordic countries. The hazardous drinking score is a composite score indicating the potential impact of drinking on health and social outcomes ranging from one (least detrimental) to five (most detrimental). It is comprised of some heavy drinking indicators, including the proportion of drinking with meals and drinking in public places (Rehm et al., 2003), all of which have been associated with more harmful outcomes for the same volume of overall drinking.

Table 1. Adult per capita consumption in different European regions, 2009

Region	Adult per capita consumption in litres of pure alcohol^a	Unrecorded per capita consumption in litres of pure alcohol	Hazardous drinking score
Central-eastern and eastern Europe	14.5 (1.7)	2.5 (0.8)	2.9 (0.3)
Central-western and western Europe	12.4 (0.8)	1.0 (0.5)	1.5 (0.9)
Nordic countries	10.4 (1.9)	1.9 (0.3)	2.8 (0.4)
Southern Europe	11.2 (1.7)	2.0 (0.5)	1.1 (0.3)
EU	12.4 (1.3)	1.6 (0.6)	1.9 (0.7)

^{a} The standard deviation is in each case indicated in the parentheses.

Source: WHO, 2012.

Fig. 3 shows the level of consumption on a country level. There are substantial differences between countries, but even the EU country with the lowest level of consumption is markedly above the global average. Country-specific figures on consumption and lifetime abstainers are presented in Annexes 1 and 2.

Unrecorded consumption makes up about 13% of all alcohol consumed in the EU (see Table 1 and the chapter on unrecorded consumption in this book). This proportion is low compared to the estimated global average of almost 30% of all alcohol consumed being unrecorded (Lachenmeier, Taylor & Rehm, 2011). What falls in the category of unrecorded consumption varies markedly between countries (for example, it consists mainly of cross-border shopping in

---

^{3} The standard drink of 12 g used here corresponds to 1 small (about 330 ml) can of beer, 1 dl of wine or one shot of spirits.

Fig. 3. Adult (15+ years) per capita alcohol consumption in litres of pure alcohol, EU countries, 2009

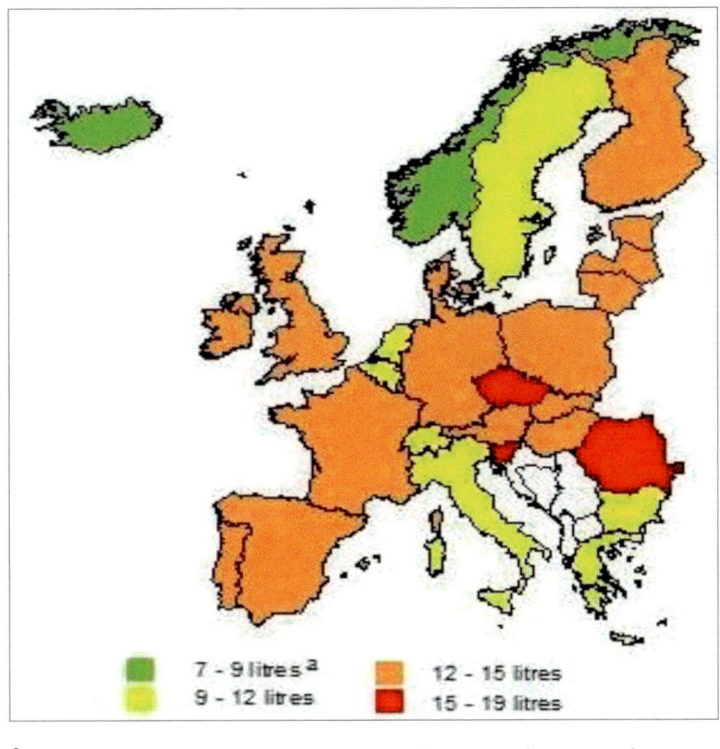

[a] Includes Malta, with 8.0 litres pure alcohol consumption per capita.

Sweden and other Nordic countries, surrogate alcohol in the Baltic countries, undeclared wine production in wine-producing countries and illegal production in some countries), and thus the health consequences are hard to assess. Based on current knowledge, however, there is no indication that unrecorded alcohol consumption has different health consequences than recorded consumption, that is, the negative consequences of unrecorded consumption are mainly due to its ethanol content and to the way in which it is consumed (see the discussion on patterns of drinking, above) (Lachenmeier et al., 2011a, 2011b).

With respect to patterns of drinking (see Table 1) and especially heavy drinking occasions, parts of Europe, particularly in the central-western and southern regions, have less of the "explosive festive drinking" style (occasional excessive drinking) than many other parts of the world (Room & Mäkelä, 2000; WHO, 2011; Rehm et al., 2004); see also Fig. 4 and Annex 3). In the Nordic countries and most of the central-eastern and eastern countries, however, irregular heavy drinking is prevalent, a pattern of drinking that has been found to be especially linked to detrimental outcomes, particularly injuries (Gmel, Kuntsche & Rehm, 2011; Landberg, 2011). The high overall volume of alcohol consumption in the EU implies that regular heavy drinking is prevalent, as also evidenced by Eurobarometer surveys (European Commission, 2010). If survey results are triangulated with the more reliable adult per capita consumption information (Rehm, Klotsche & Patra, 2007; Rehm et al., 2010a), it is estimated that 4.6% of men and 0.1% of women drink more than 5 standard drinks of 12 g on average every day.

Trends in alcohol consumption

The only indicator that allows reliable tracking of alcohol consumption over time is recorded adult per capita consumption, as this information is available on a yearly basis in all EU countries.

Fig. 4. Global patterns of drinking, 2005

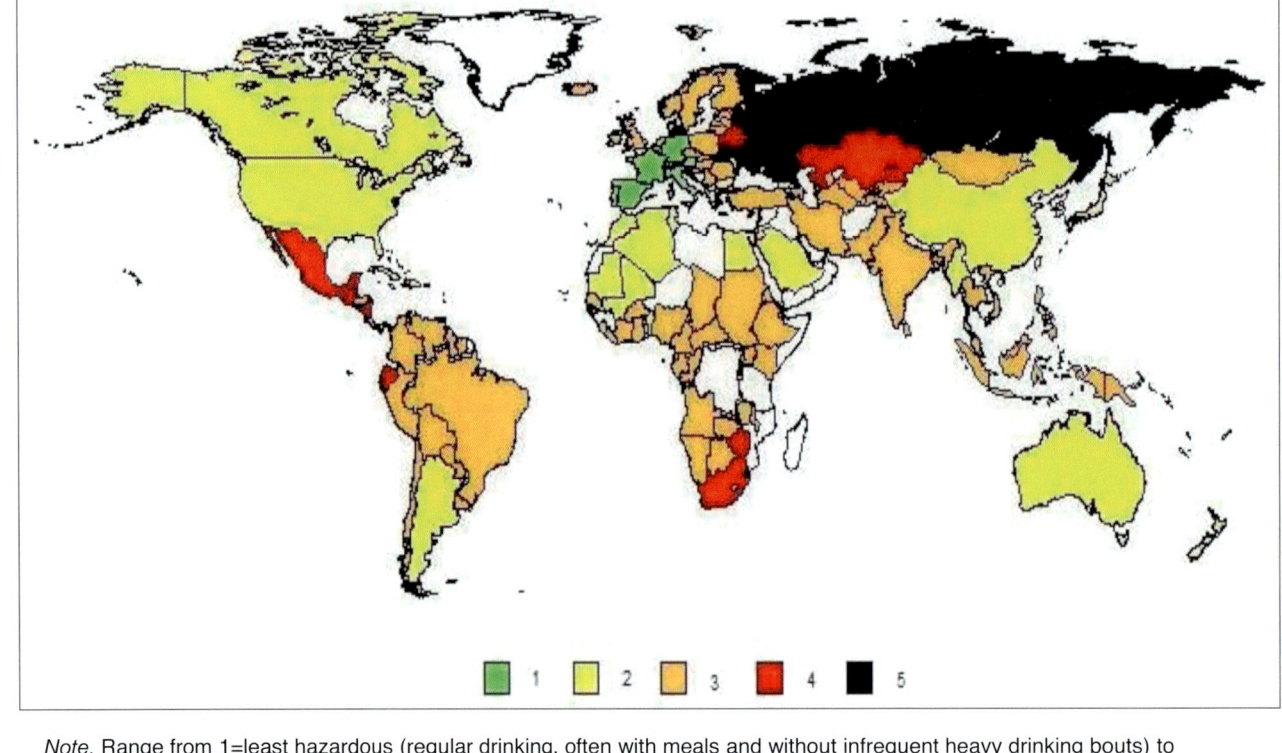

Note. Range from 1=least hazardous (regular drinking, often with meals and without infrequent heavy drinking bouts) to 5= most hazardous (infrequent but heavy drinking outside of meals).

As shown in Fig. 5a, recorded adult per capita consumption has been stable over the past 10 years for the EU as a whole, with minimal changes both in the overall level of consumption and in the beverage-specific trends, although there have been varying trends in the different regions (Figs. 5b–e).

Fig. 5a. Adult per capita alcohol consumption in the EU since 2000

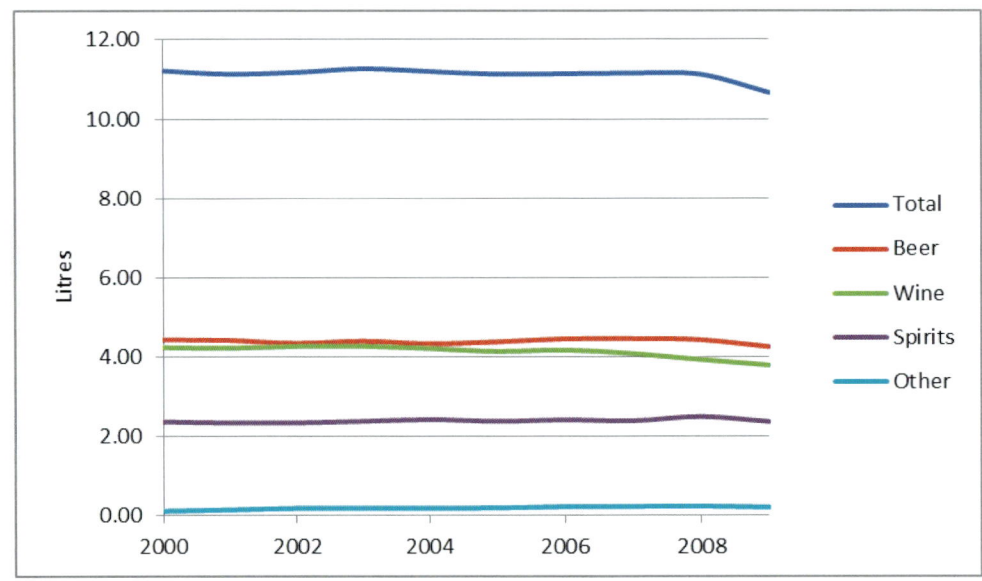

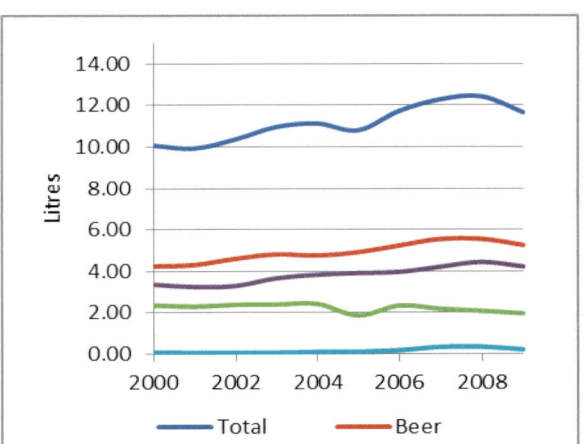

Fig. 5b. Adult per capita alcohol consumption in central-east and eastern Europe since 2000

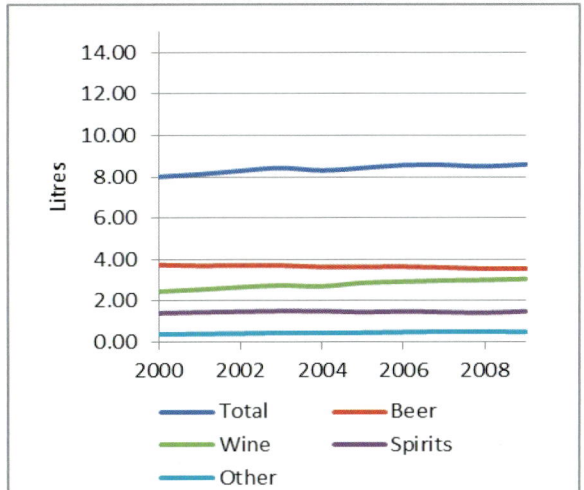

Fig. 5c. Adult per capita alcohol consumption in the Nordic countries since 2000

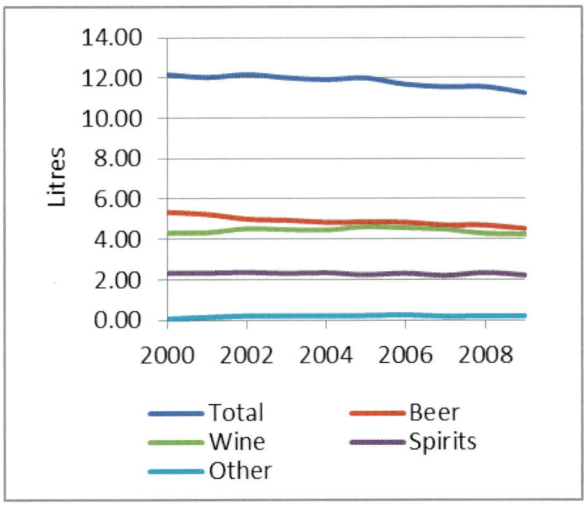

Fig. 5d. Adult per capita alcohol consumption in central-west and western Europe since 2000

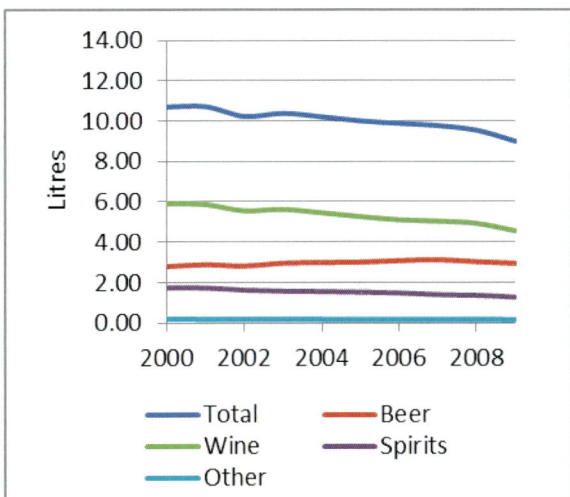

Fig. 5e. Adult per capita consumption in southern Europe since 2000

Although the European per capita consumption of alcohol has remained nearly constant over the past decade, this apparent steadiness hides two opposing trends. The Nordic countries and eastern Europe have seen an increase in adult per capita consumption, whereas western and southern Europe have experienced a decrease. Beer is the most prominent alcoholic beverage in almost all regions. Only in southern Europe does wine remain the most frequently consumed alcoholic drink, but even in southern Europe, the consumption of wine has been decreasing at a high rate whereas beer consumption is only rising slightly. This decrease in wine intake is mainly responsible for the strong downward trend in total alcohol consumption in southern Europe. The Nordic countries are moving in the opposite direction to the southern countries, although the changes are not as marked: wine consumption has steadily increased in the past decade while beer has lost some of its popularity. Southern and eastern Europe are the two regions that show the largest amount of change in their total alcohol consumption, but these changes tend to cancel each other out and are not reflected in the EU average.

Alcohol-attributable burden of disease in Europe

The relationship between alcohol consumption and disease and injury

Many categories of disease have names which indicate that alcohol is an essential cause and that 100% of the incidence of these diseases is attributable to alcohol. While alcohol-use disorders such as alcohol dependence and the harmful use of alcohol as defined by the International Classification of Disease (ICD-10) (WHO, 1992) are certainly the most important of these categories, they are not the only ones by far. Rehm and colleagues listed more than 40 such conditions recorded in the ICD-10, ranging from chronic disease (such as K70 alcoholic liver disease or K86.0 alcohol-induced chronic pancreatitis) to injury (such as X45 accidental poisoning by and exposure to alcohol) to the drinking of a pregnant woman harming the fetus (for example, Q86.0 fetal alcohol syndrome) (Rehm et al., 2010a).

There are, however, even more conditions where alcohol is a component cause (Rothman, Greenland & Lash, 2008), meaning that not all such diseases are caused by alcohol but if there was no consumption of alcohol, some instances of these conditions would not have occurred. If traffic injury mortality is taken as an example, many influencing causal factors are seen such as road conditions, traffic density or the wearing of seat belts. In a certain fraction of these deaths, alcohol consumption has been causal, that is, without drinking, these deaths would never have happened.

Box 1 provides an overview of conditions where alcohol has been determined to be causal, and of conditions that could be modelled in this analysis because of the availability of data.

Box 1. Alcohol-attributable disease and injury 2005 (green mainly protective)

Chronic and infectious disease

Cancer: nasopharyngeal, oesophageal, laryngeal, liver, colon/rectal, female breast
Neuropsychiatric diseases: alcohol use disorders (100% alcohol-attributable), primary epilepsy
Diabetes
Cardiovascular diseases: hypertensive diseases, ischaemic heart disease, ischaemic stroke, hemorrhagic stroke, cardiac arrhythmias
Gastrointestinal diseases: liver cirrhosis, pancreatitis
Infectious diseases: tuberculosis, effect of alcohol on course of HIV/AIDS, lower respiratory infections
Conditions arising during perinatal period: low birth weight, fetal alcohol syndrome (100% alcohol-attributable, no available data for this report)

Injury

Unintentional injury: transport injuries, falls, drowning, fire, poisonings, exposure to forces of nature, other unintentional injuries
Intentional injury: self-inflicted injuries, interpersonal violence, other intentional injuries

---

The problem of time lag

In most analyses of the alcohol-attributable burden on health, the calculations are conducted as if the health consequences of alcohol consumption are immediate. While it is true that for most of the alcohol-attributable health burden, even with respect to chronic diseases such as cirrhosis, a large part of the effects due to changes in alcohol consumption can be seen immediately at the population level (Leon et al., 1997; Holmes et al., 2011; Zatonski et al., 2010), cancer is different. The effect of alcohol consumption on cancer can only be seen years later (often as long as two decades). For the purpose of illustrating the entire alcohol-attributable burden, however, cancer deaths are included here, especially given that in Europe 1 in 10 cancers in men and 1 in 33 cancers in women were found to be alcohol-related in a recent large study (Schütze et al., 2011). In interpreting the effect of alcohol, it should be borne in mind that this assumes uniform exposure to alcohol for at least the previous two decades.

Alcohol-attributable mortality in Europe

Figs. 6–8 provide an overview of alcohol-attributable mortality, showing both the number of deaths and potential years of life lost due to premature mortality in the group aged 15–64 years. The older age groups are not included as death certificates become more problematic for older people (Harteloh, de Bruin & Kardaun, 2010), especially for the very old (Alpérovitch et al., 2009), and as the relative risks for alcohol-attributable causes tend to go down with age (Klatsky & Udaltsova, 2007) so that both the detrimental and the beneficial consequences of consumption tend to be exaggerated in the older age group. The group aged under 15 years is also excluded, since alcohol-attributable deaths in this group are very rare except as the result of the impact of someone else's drinking (for example, traffic fatalities caused by drunk drivers; this will be reported in the section "Health harm to others due to alcohol consumption", below).

Number of deaths and standardized mortality rates due to alcohol consumption

It is estimated that 94 451 men and 25 284 women aged between 15 and 64 years died of alcohol-attributable causes in the EU in 2004 (total 119 735). This corresponds to 13.9% of all deaths in men and 7.7% of all deaths in women in this age category (11.8% of all deaths). Figs. 6 and 7 provide an overview of details by region and by country, as well as of standardized mortality rates.

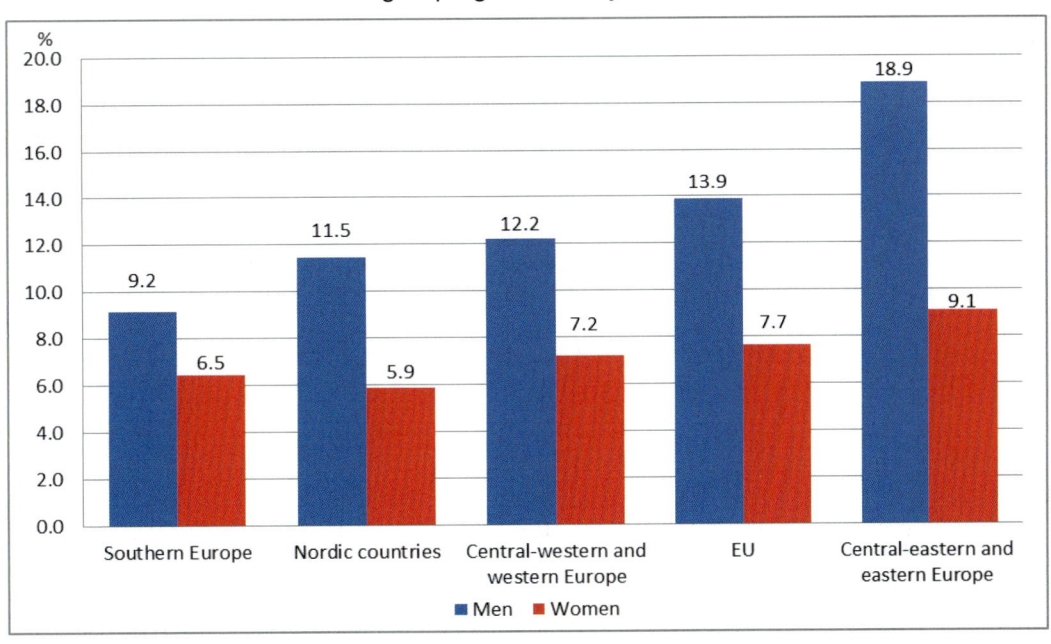

Fig. 6. Regional variations in proportion of alcohol-attributable deaths to all deaths in the group aged 15–64 years, 2004

The proportions of alcohol-attributable deaths to all deaths show some variation (Fig. 6). The estimate of 11.8% of mortality being caused by alcohol signals a high level of overall burden, and even in the region with the relatively lowest burden, southern Europe, about 9.2% and 6.5% of all deaths in men and women, respectively, are due to alcohol. This means that in the European region which has the lowest alcohol-attributable burden, more than 1 in every 11 male deaths and 1 in every 16 female deaths are due to alcohol.

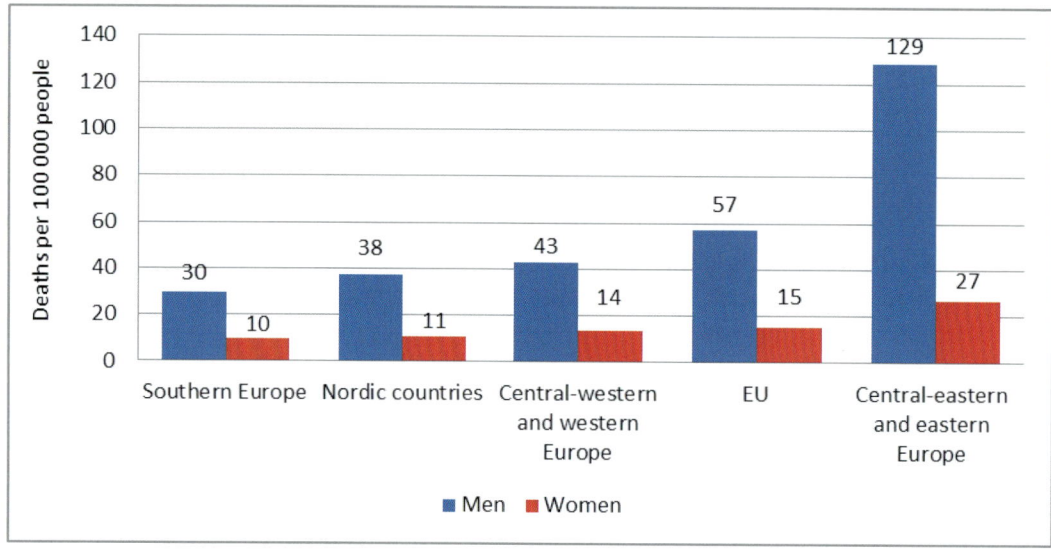

Fig. 7. Regional variations in standardized mortality attributable to alcohol per 100 000, by sex in the group aged 15–64 years, 2004

Fig. 7 shows the standardized alcohol-attributable mortality rates by region. As expected, the mortality rate is much lower among women compared to men. These sex differences are less pronounced in the proportion of deaths attributable to alcohol consumption, because in the group aged 15–64 years mortality is generally higher in men. Regional variations are also more marked, about threefold for women and almost fivefold for men.

Countries in central-eastern and eastern Europe have the highest rate of alcohol-attributable deaths for both sexes: in men this is more than twice the rate of the EU as a whole (57 vs. 129 deaths per 100 000), and in women it is almost twice (15 vs. 27 deaths per 100 000). In interpreting the numbers, it should be remembered that alcohol consumption in the southern European countries has markedly decreased over recent decades, so that their cancer rates are overestimated, while there are no such tendencies in the other parts of Europe.

Fig. 8 provides an overview of the proportions of alcohol-attributable deaths to all deaths at the country level.

The separation between regions is relatively clear, especially for men. However, different countries rank highest for the alcohol-attributable burden within central-eastern and eastern Europe when men and women are considered separately. For men, the highest rates are in the Baltic countries of Estonia and Lithuania, where more than 25% of deaths are attributable to alcohol, whereas for women, the highest burden is in Romania. At the other end of the spectrum, the islands of Cyprus and Malta show the relatively lowest burden of alcohol-attributable mortality.

Fig. 8. Country variations in the proportion of alcohol-attributable deaths to all deaths in the group aged 15–64 years for women (left) and men (right), 2004

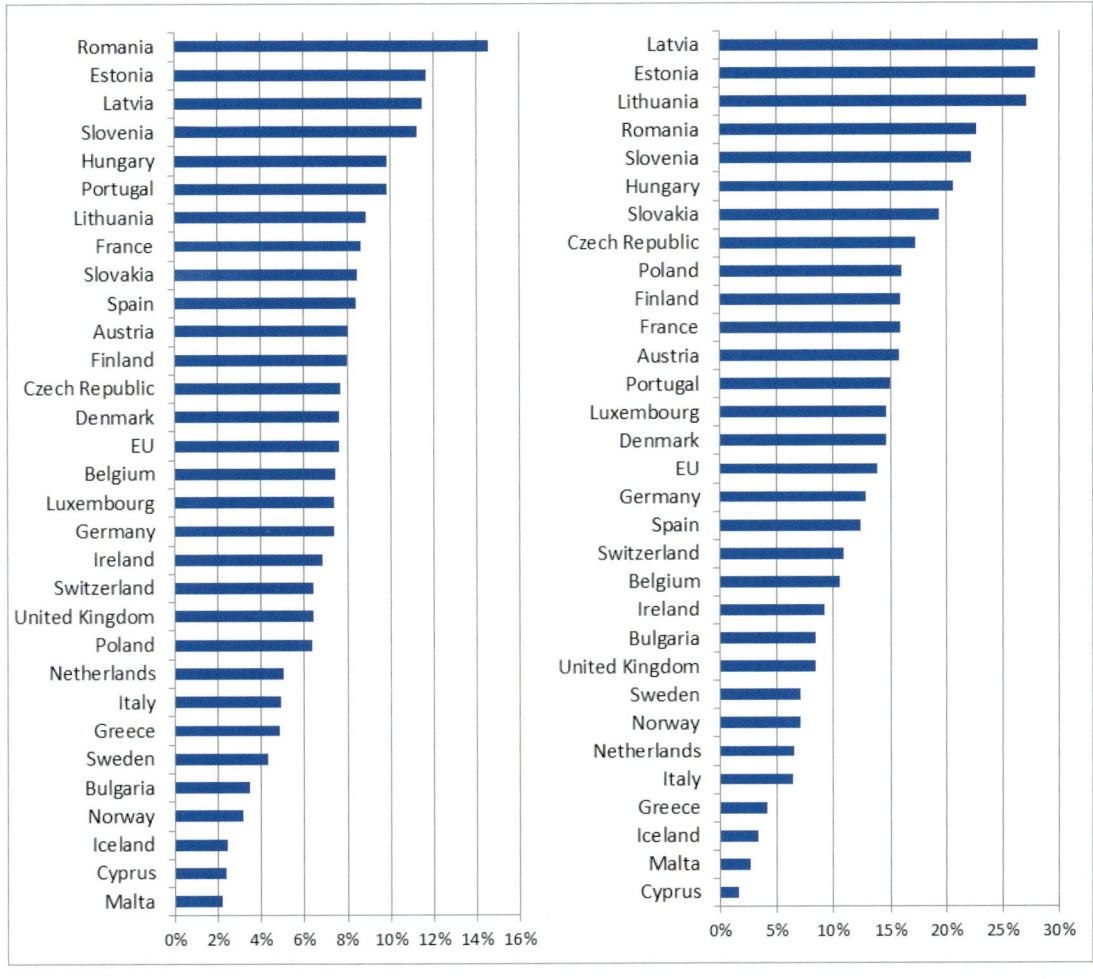

Note. The calculation for Latvia was made from initial data received from the survey, which were later revised. The initial data were higher than the second set of data.

So far, only alcohol-attributable deaths have been considered as a proportion of all-cause mortality. Table 2 provides an overview of alcohol-attributable deaths in Europe by broad disease categories, separating the detrimental and protective influences. The distribution varies markedly by sex and region (for the latter see below). For men, the highest contribution to alcohol-attributable mortality is made by liver cirrhosis (26%) and unintentional injury (23%), followed by cancer (16%) and intentional injury (15%). For women, more than two thirds of alcohol-attributable deaths arise from liver cirrhosis (37%) and cancer (31%) (the largest proportion of which concerns breast cancer, with 21%), with cardiovascular disease other than ischaemic heart disease as a distant third cause (11%). The beneficial effects of alcohol consumption in terms of mortality are primarily observed with respect to ischaemic heart disease in men (98%). In contrast, one third of these beneficial effects in women are observed in other disease categories (such as diabetes, but mainly cardiovascular diseases other than ischaemic heart disease, hypertensive diseases and ischaemic stroke).

In all regions, alcohol-attributable deaths in men are distributed more evenly between the above-mentioned broad disease categories than is observed for women. Whereas for men no category has more than 33% of all alcohol-attributable deaths, for women the top two disease categories in all regions and in the EU are above 60%, and in two of the four regions they are over 70%.

Table 2. Alcohol-attributable deaths in Europe by broad disease categories in the group aged 15–64 years, 2004

Effects	Men	Women	Men (%)	Women (%)
Detrimental effects				
Cancer	17 358	8 668	15.9	30.7
Cardiovascular diseases other than ischaemic heart disease	7 914	3 127	7.2	11.1
Mental and neurological disorders	10 868	2 330	9.9	8.3
Liver cirrhosis	28 449	10 508	26.0	37.2
Unintentional injury	24 912	1 795	22.8	6.4
Intentional injury	16 562	1 167	15.1	4.1
Other detrimental	3 455	637	3.2	2.3
Total detrimental	109 517	28 232	100.0	100.0
Beneficial effects				
Ischaemic heart disease	14 736	1 800	97.8	61.1
Other beneficial	330	1 147	2.2	38.9
Total beneficial	15 065	2 947	100.0	100.0

There is considerable variation between regions. Cardiovascular diseases (other than ischaemic heart disease) and injuries are proportionately higher in central-eastern and eastern Europe, which is a reflection of the combination of high overall volume combined with irregular heavy drinking occasions (Gmel, Kuntsche & Rehm, 2011; Rehm et al., 2007). Mental and neurological disorders are proportionately higher in the Nordic countries, reflecting the relatively high prevalence of alcohol dependence and alcohol-use disorders in this region. Cancer is proportionately higher in southern Europe, which reflects the much higher levels of consumption prevalent two decades ago (WHO, 2011); (see Rehm et al. (2011) for more details). As indicated above, cancer takes a long time to develop. The category which has the most similar relative proportion across the regions is liver cirrhosis, varying between 23.3% and 28.4% for men and 31.0% and 39.9% for women.

Fig. 9 provides an overview of the proportions of specific disease categories which are alcohol-attributable.

Alcohol causes between 75% and 80% of all liver cirrhosis in Europe. This can be attributed to a relatively low prevalence of other risk factors for this disease in Europe and, as a consequence, trends in liver cirrhosis mortality rates closely follow trends in alcohol consumption (see (Zatonski et al. (2010) for a general overview, and Leon & McCambridge (2006) for an example in Great Britain). Alcohol-attributable proportions were estimated using alcohol-attributable fractions for all liver cirrhosis based on exposure and the relative risks (Rehm et al., 2010b), rather than using records of the proportions of deaths indicating alcoholic liver cirrhosis as one of the causes of death. The reason for this procedure is as follows. First, based on death certificates, the proportion of liver cirrhosis attributable to alcohol is often underestimated (Puffer & Griffith, 1967; Haberman & Weinbaum, 1990) for various reasons including stigma and potential insurance problems. Second, it has long been recognized that when detailed causes of death categories are indicated on death certificates, there is a higher degree of misclassification of the causes of death. Thus, the misclassification associated with the combined category of liver cirrhosis should be smaller than the misclassification for different subcategories such as alcoholic liver cirrhosis.

Fig. 9. Proportion of deaths within major disease categories attributable to alcohol in the EU for the group aged 15–64 years, 2004

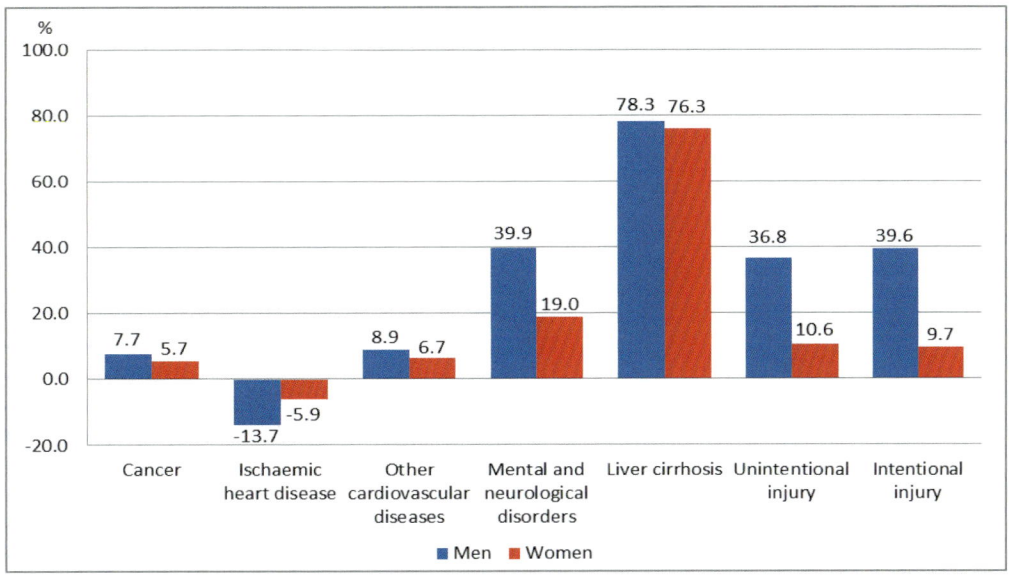

With respect to the other proportions, a marked impact of alcohol consumption on cancer mortality was observed well in line with the results of the largest cohort study on alcohol and cancer in this region (Schütze et al., 2011); on mortality from cardiovascular diseases other than heart disease (for the latter an overall cardioprotective effect was observed; see Puddey et al., 1999; Rehm, Sempos & Trevisan, 2003); and on injury, both unintentional and intentional. The effect on mental health and neurological disorders is due mainly to alcohol dependence, which is more prevalent in Europe than in most other parts of the world (Rehm et al., 2009; Wittchen et al., 2011).

Alcohol-attributable burden of disease and standardized rates of DALYs due to alcohol

DALYs are a summary measure of health which adds potential years of life lost and years lived with disability, that is, DALYs comprise all years of life lost due to premature mortality and due to living with disability. In 2004, an estimated 3 359 000 DALYs in men and 684 000 DALYs in women were lost due to alcohol-attributable causes in the group aged 15–64 years in the EU (total 4 043 000). This corresponds to 15.2% of all DALYs in men and 3.9% of all DALYs in women (10.2% of all DALYs). Figs. 10–12 provide an overview of details by region and country, as well as of standardized mortality rates.

The differences between the two regions with the lowest and the highest proportions of alcohol-attributable DALYs in both sexes are more than twofold: in southern Europe the proportions are 8% in men and 2% in women, while in central-eastern and eastern Europe they are 20% in men and 5% in women. A look at individual countries reveals a greater variation, but most of the variations occur between regions. In central-eastern and eastern Europe (the region with the highest alcohol-attributable burden of disease), Bulgaria has the lowest alcohol-attributable burden for both men and women (Fig. 11). The Nordic countries display the greatest variation in alcohol-attributable burden of disease within a region, with Norway and Sweden among the European countries with the highest proportion for women while Finland and Norway are among those with the highest proportion for men. Countries in central-western and western Europe all cluster around the EU mean, and the southern European countries are all among the countries with lower burdens (see Fig. 11).

Alcohol in the European Union
page 22

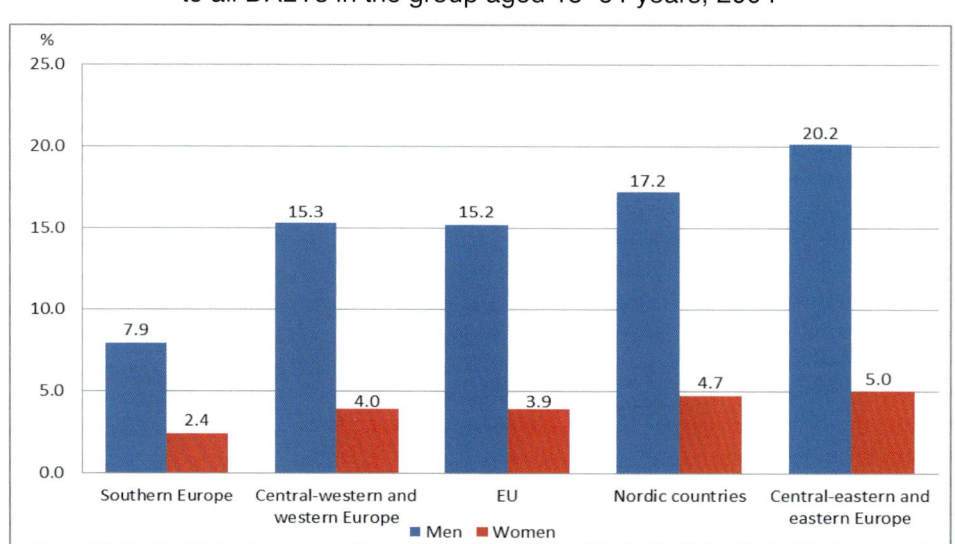

Fig. 10. Regional variation in the proportion of alcohol-attributable DALYs to all DALYs in the group aged 15–64 years, 2004

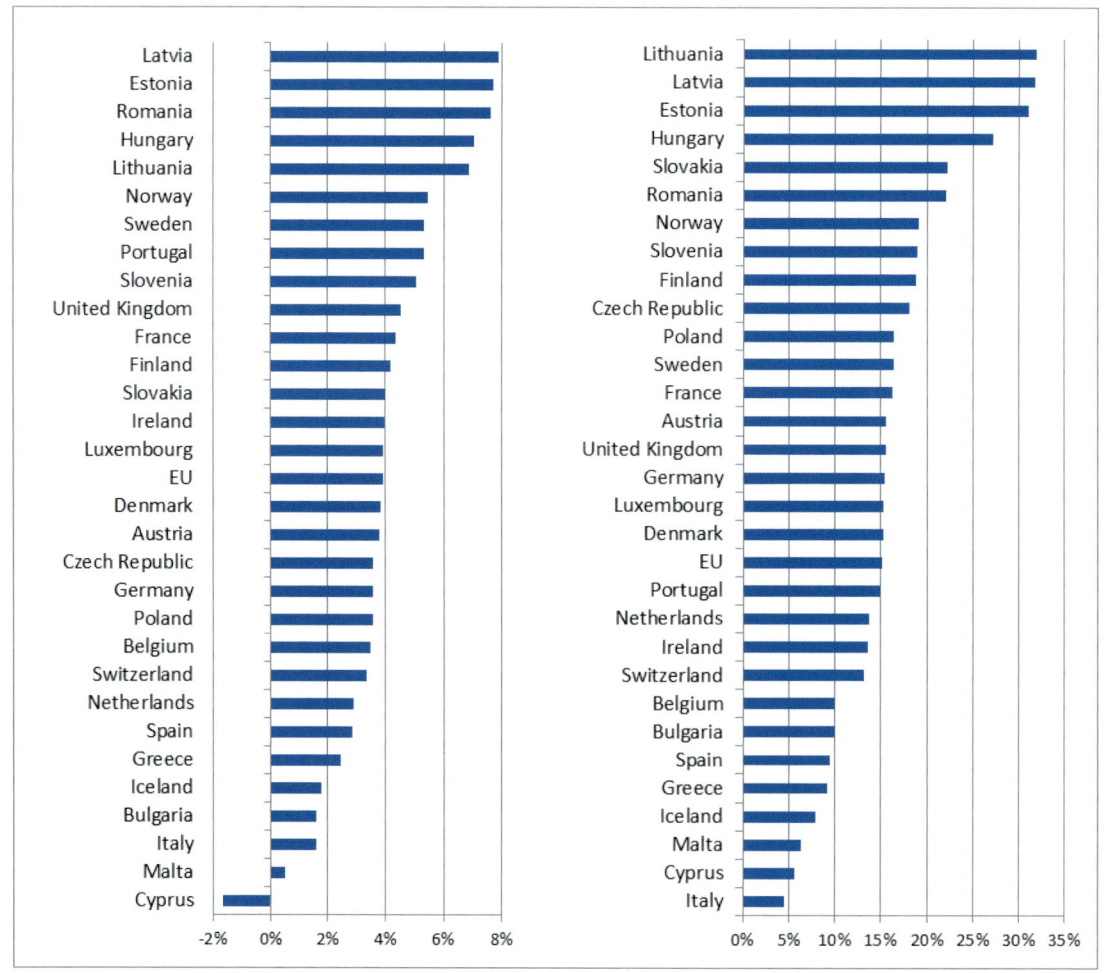

Fig. 11. Country variations in the percentage of alcohol-attributable DALYs to all DALYs in the group aged 15–64 years, women (left) and men (right), 2004

Note. The calculations for Latvia were made from initial data received from the survey, which were later revised. The initial data were higher than the second set of data.

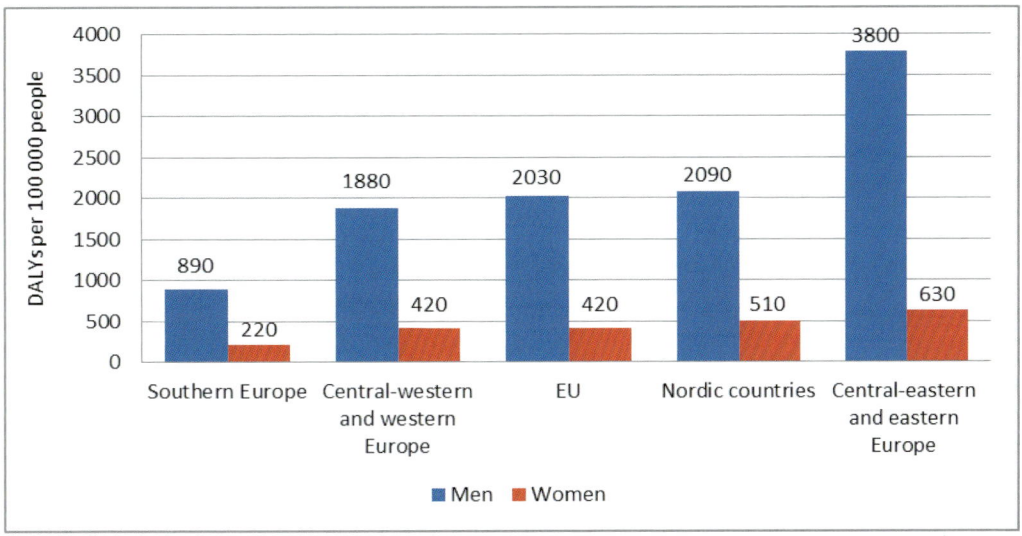

Fig. 12. Regional variation of standardized DALY rates per 100 000 by sex in the group aged 15–64 years, 2004

The Nordic countries show higher rates of alcohol-attributable DALYs overall due to their relatively higher (compared to other European regions) rates of years lived with disability (details not shown). For both men and women, the standardized rates of alcohol-attributable DALYs in the Nordic countries are above the EU average (Fig. 12), an observation which fits well with the results of time-series modelling where the effects of alcohol per unit consumed were higher in the Nordic countries compared to central-western, western and southern countries. The central-eastern and eastern countries have not been included in previous analyses (see Norström, 2001), mainly due to the effects of alcohol on injury, both intentional and unintentional (Skog, 2001; Rossow, 2001; Ramstedt, 2001). Substantial country variations in standardized DALY rates are only observed within the Nordic countries.

Table 3 provides an overview of the main causes of the alcohol-attributable burden of disease, which is markedly different from the distribution of the main causes of alcohol-attributable mortality. Mental and neurological disorders comprise the largest proportion of the alcohol-attributable burden of disease (as measured in DALYs) for both men (46%) and women (44%). For men, injuries are the second largest contributor to the burden of disease (unintentional 17%; intentional 10%), whereas for women liver cirrhosis is the second largest contributor (25%). The high burden of mental and neurological disorders is almost entirely due to alcohol-use disorders, especially alcohol dependence. Alcohol-use disorders are much less fatal compared to other alcohol-related diseases such as cancer and cardiovascular diseases, thus they contribute relatively more to the alcohol-attributable burden of disease than to alcohol-attributable mortality.

Harm to other people's health due to alcohol consumption

So far the effects of alcohol consumption on the mortality of and burden of disease on drinkers themselves have been discussed. Drinkers not only endanger their own health, however, but also the health of others (for example, drinking during pregnancy may risk the health of the newborn; drinking shortly before or while driving may cause injury or death to others). This section describes the major harm to other people's health arising from alcohol consumption. Such harm is borne by people who may or may not drink, but it is caused by other people's drinking (for example, motor vehicle accident deaths to passengers and other drivers and road-users

Table 3. Alcohol-attributable burden of disease in DALYs in Europe by broad disease categories in the group aged 15–64 years, 2004

Effects	Men	Women	Men (%)	Women (%)
Detrimental effects				
Cancer	251 891	151 671	6.9	17.5
Cardiovascular diseases other than ischaemic heart disease	128 336	25 969	3.5	3.0
Mental and neurological disorders	1 691 310	382 584	46.3	44.2
Liver cirrhosis	512 560	212 676	14.0	24.6
Unintentional Injury	634 959	50 936	17.4	5.9
Intentional injury	347 225	24 147	9.5	2.8
Other detrimental	83 640	18 149	2.3	2.1
Total detrimental	3 649 921	866 131	100.00	100.00
Beneficial effects				
Ischaemic heart disease	275 588	87 887	94.8	48.3
Other beneficial	15 049	94 054	5.2	51.7
Total beneficial	290 637	181 941	100.0	100.0

attributable to the drinking of a drunk driver; low birth weight caused by a mother drinking during pregnancy; homicide and violence caused by a person who has been drinking). Although an individual's drinking plays a role in the probability that he/she will be assaulted, for this report mortality and morbidity attributable to violence because of the drinking of others were calculated based solely on the drinking of others and did not incorporate the effects of drinking by the individual who was assaulted. Additionally, as harm to others affects people of all ages, this analysis will not be restricted to people in a particular age group, as was the case in the main analysis which examined alcohol-related harm (not including harm to others) in people aged 15–64 years.

In the EU in 2004, for men of all ages, 5564 deaths, 139 824 potential years of life lost, 18 987 years lived with disability and 158 811 DALYs were attributable to harm to others caused by alcohol consumption; for women of all ages the figures were 2146 deaths, 51 326 potential years of life lost, 8423 years lived with disability and 59 749 DALYs (totals of 7710 deaths, 191 151 potential years of life lost, 27 410 years lived with disability and 218 560 DALYs). Table 4 outlines the alcohol-attributable burden on health in the EU in 2004 caused by harm to others. The main alcohol-attributable cause of harm to others was transport injuries, with violence being a distant second cause. The observations of the proportionate roles played by transport injuries, violence and low birth weight in alcohol-attributable harm to others are similar to those from Australia in 2005 where, in total, 367 people died due to alcohol consumption by others: 75.4% from motor vehicle accidents, 21.0% from assaults, and 3.6% from fetal alcohol syndrome which included low birth weight (Laslett et al., 2010). Fetal alcohol syndrome mortality percentages are higher in Australia when compared to low birth weight mortality percentages in the EU, as fetal alcohol syndrome data from Australia include additional causes of death and disability that are not included in this report due to the limitations of mortality data at an international level.

Figs. 13 and 14 outline the relative burden arising from harm to others as measured by the number of deaths and DALYs attributable to alcohol consumption at a regional level. In the EU in 2004, 3.3% of the total burden measured in deaths (3.1% for men; 3.8% for women) and 4.5% of the total burden measured in DALYS (4.0% for men; 6.9% for women) were due to alcohol-attributable harm to others. Women carried a higher percentage of the total alcohol-attributable burden as measured in deaths caused by harm to others compared to men, apart from in southern Europe.

Table 4. Alcohol-attributable mortality and burden of disease in the EU caused by harm to others in the group aged 15–64 years, 2004

Causes of deaths and DALYs	Men	Women	Men (%)	Women (%)
Deaths				
Low birth weight	62	45	1.1	2.1
Violence	1 586	685	28.5	31.9
Transport injuries	3 916	1 416	70.4	66.0
Total	5 564	2 147	100.0	100.0
DALYs				
Low birth weight	2 685	2 063	1.7	3.5
Violence	47 956	18 967	30.2	31.7
Transport injuries	108 170	38 719	68.1	64.8
Total	158 811	59 749	100.0	100.0

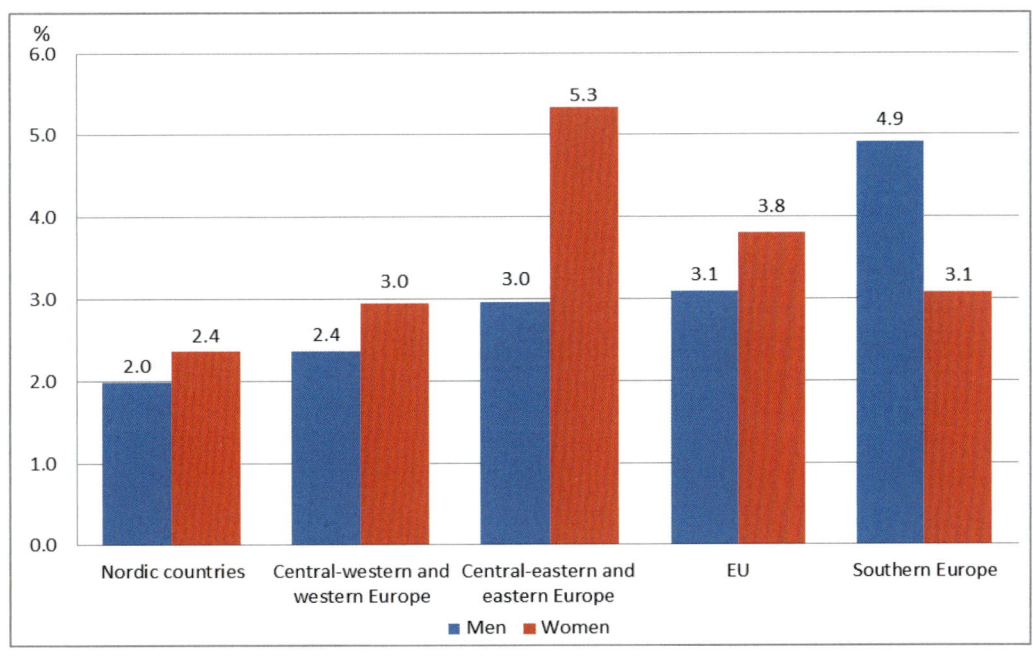

Fig. 13. Proportion of deaths attributable to alcohol consumption caused by harm to others by European region in the group aged 15–64 years, 2004

Southern Europe experiences the greatest proportion of alcohol-attributable harm to others when compared to total alcohol-attributable harm for that region as measured by deaths. This is in comparison to central-eastern and eastern Europe, where calculations indicate high alcohol-attributable fractions for motor vehicle accidents where the drunk driver harms himself. Thus specific relative risks for central-east and eastern Europe are required to accurately characterize the alcohol-attributable fraction for drunk drivers harming themselves and alcohol-attributable fraction for drunk drivers harming others. In addition, the high mortality rate due to alcohol-attributable causes other than motor vehicle accidents, assaults, and low birth weight in central-eastern and eastern Europe lowers those regions' proportion of alcohol-attributable deaths due to harm to others to all alcohol-attributable deaths. In contrast, this latter proportion is higher in southern Europe, where the alcohol-attributable mortality rate is much lower. These estimates of alcohol-attributable harm to others are limited to the health outcomes of mortality and disability and do not include the other areas of harm, namely: crime and public disorder, workplace injuries and opportunity costs, and the social impact on the drinker's family and social networks.

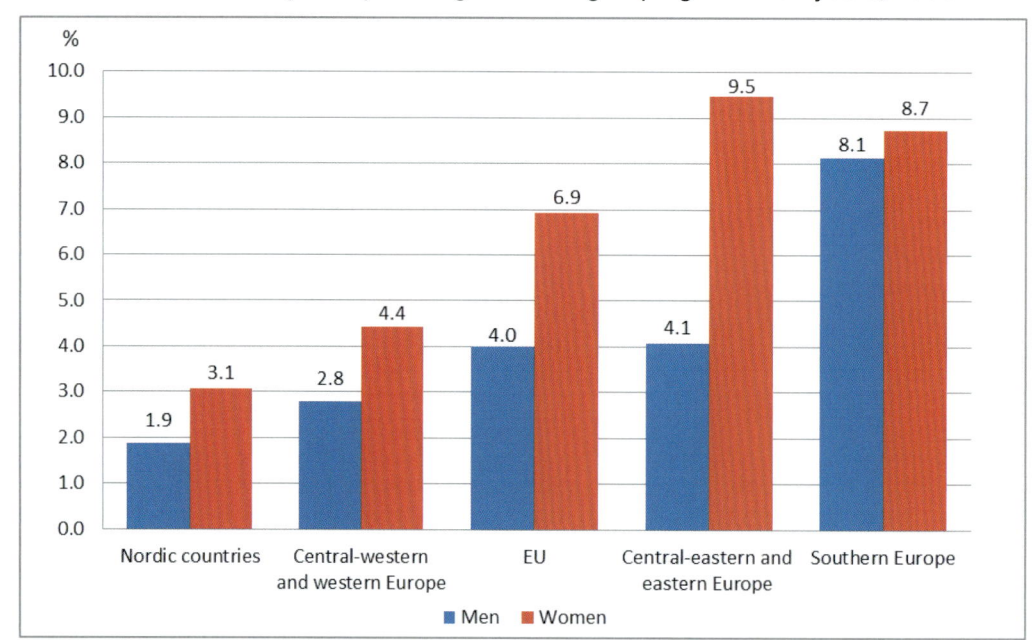

Fig. 14. Proportion of DALYs attributable to alcohol consumption caused by harm to others by European region in the group aged 15–64 years, 2004

Conclusions

Alcohol consumption in the EU is giving rise to a considerable health burden. Additionally, there are huge social and economic burdens resulting from the effects of alcohol consumption on individuals, families, work and society. Many of these resulting burdens fall upon people other than the drinker, and while full quantification of the harm to others is difficult, the data available for Europe suggest that there is a large impact. In theory, all alcohol-related burdens on health are avoidable.

References

Alpérovitch A et al. (2009). Do we really know the cause of death of the very old? Comparison between official mortality statistics and cohort study classification. *European Journal of Epidemiology*, 24:669–675.

Anderson P, Baumberg B (2006). *Alcohol in Europe. A public health perspective*. London, Institute of Alcohol Studies (http://ec.europa.eu/health-eu/doc/alcoholineu_content_en.pdf, accessed 18 February 2012).

European Commission (2010). *EU citizens' attitudes towards alcohol. Special Eurobarometer 331*. Brussels, European Commission.

Gmel G, Kuntsche E, Rehm J (2011). Risky single occasion drinking: bingeing is not bingeing. *Addiction*, 106:1037–1045.

Gmel G, Rehm J (2004). Measuring alcohol consumption. *Contemporary Drug Problems*, 31(3):467–540.

Groves RM (2004). *Survey errors and survey costs*. Chichester, John Wiley and Sons Ltd. (Wiley Series in Survey Methodology).

Haberman PW, Weinbaum DF (1990). Liver cirrhosis with and without mention of alcohol as cause of death. *British Journal of Addiction*, 85:217–222.

Harteloh P, de Bruin K, Kardaun J (2010). The reliability of cause-of-death coding in the Netherlands. *European Journal of Epidemiology*, 25:531–538.

Holmes J et al. (2011). *Time lags in the effects of alcohol policy interventions*. 37th Annual Alcohol Epidemiology Symposium of the Kettil Bruun Society, Melbourne, 11–15 April 2011.

Iontchev A (1998). Central and Eastern Europe. In: Grant M, ed. *Alcohol and emerging markets: patterns, problems, and responses*. Washington, DC, International Center for Alcohol Policies.

Klatsky AL, Udaltsova N (2007). Alcohol drinking and total mortality risk. *Annals of Epidemiology*, 17:S63–S67.

Lachenmeier DW et al. (2011a). Quality of illegally and informally produced alcohol in Europe: results from the AMPHORA project. *Adicciones*, 23:133–140.

Lachenmeier DW et al. (2011b). Is contaminated unrecorded alcohol a health problem in the European Union? A review of existing and methodological outline for future studies. *Addiction*, 106:20–30.

Lachenmeier DW, Taylor BJ, Rehm J (2011). Alcohol under the radar: do we have policy options regarding unrecorded alcohol? *International Journal of Drug Policy*, 22:153–160.

Landberg J (2011). Self-reported alcohol consumption and the risk of alcohol-related problems: a comparative risk-curve analysis of the 3 Baltic countries, Sweden, and Italy. *Alcoholism: Clinical and Experimental Research*, 36(1):113–118.

Laslett AM et al. (2010). *The range and magnitude of alcohol's harm to others*. Fitzroy, VIC, Turning Point Alcohol & Drug Centre, Eastern Health.

Leifman H (2002). Trends in popular drinking. In: Norström T, ed. *Alcohol in postwar Europe: consumption, drinking patterns, consequences and policy responses in 15 European countries*. Stockholm, National Institute of Public Health and Almqvist & Wiksell International.

Leon D et al. (1997). Huge variation in Russian mortality rates 1984-1994: artefact, alcohol, or what? *Lancet*, 350:383–388.

Leon DA, McCambridge J (2006). Liver cirrhosis mortality rates in Britain from 1950 to 2002: an analysis of routine data. *Lancet*, 367:52–56.

Mäkelä P et al. (2001). Episodic heavy drinking in four Nordic countries: a comparative survey. *Addiction*, 96(11):1575–1588.

McGovern PE (2007). *Ancient wine*. Princeton, NJ, Princeton University Press.

Norström T (2001). Per capita alcohol consumption and all-cause mortality in 14 European countries. *Addiction*, 96:S113–S128.

Phillips R (2000). *A short history of wine*. New York, NY, Harper Collins.

Popova S et al. (2007). Comparing alcohol consumption in central and eastern Europe to other European countries. *Alcohol and Alcoholism*, 42(5):465–473.

Puddey IB, Rakic V, Dimmitt SB (1999). Influence of pattern of drinking on cardiovascular disease and cardiovascular risk factors – a review. *Addiction*, 94:649–663.

Puffer RR, Griffith GW (1967). *Patterns of urban mortality: report of the Inter-American Investigation of Mortality*. Washington, DC, Pan American Health Organization.

Ramstedt M (2001). Alcohol and suicide in 14 European countries. *Addiction*, 96:59S–75S.

Rehm J et al. (2003). The global distribution of average volume of alcohol consumption and patterns of drinking. *European Addiction Research*, 9:147–156.

Rehm J et al. (2004). Alcohol use. In: Ezzati M, Lopez AD, Rodgers A, Murray CJL, eds. *Comparative quantification of health risks: global and regional burden of disease attributable to selected major risk factors, Vol. 1*. Geneva, World Health Organization:959–1109.

Rehm J et al. (2007). Alcohol accounts for a high proportion of premature mortality in central and eastern Europe. *International Journal of Epidemiology*, 36:458–467.

Rehm J et al. (2009). Global burden of disease and injury and economic cost attributable to alcohol use and alcohol use disorders. *Lancet,* 373:2223–2233.

Rehm J et al. (2010a). Statistical modeling of volume of alcohol exposure for epidemiological studies of population health: the example of the US. *Population Health Metrics,* 8:3.

Rehm J et al. (2010b). Alcohol as a risk factor for liver cirrhosis – a systematic review and meta-analysis. *Drug and Alcohol Review,* 29:437–445.

Rehm J, Klotsche J, Patra J (2007). Comparative quantification of alcohol exposure as risk factor for global burden of disease. *International Journal of Methods in Psychiatric Research,* 16:66–76.

Rehm J, Sempos C, Trevisan M (2003). Average volume of alcohol consumption, patterns of drinking and risk of coronary heart disease – a review. *Journal of Cardiovascular Risk,* 10:15–20.

Rehm J, Zatonski W, Taylor B (2011). Epidemiology and alcohol policy in Europe. *Addiction,* 106 (Suppl.1):11–19.

Room R, Mäkelä K (2000). Typologies of the cultural position of drinking. *Journal of Studies on Alcohol,* 61(3):475–483.

Room R (1992). The impossible dream? Routes to reducing alcohol problems in a temperance culture. *Journal of Substance Abuse,* 4(1):91–106.

Room R (2010). Alkogol'naya politika: polozhenie del i problemy v Evrope i Severnoi Azii [Alcohol politics: status of the problem in Europe and North Asia]. In: Khalturnia DA, Korotaev AV, eds. *Alkogol'naya katastrofa i vozmozhnosti gosudarstvennoi politiki v preodolenii alkogol'noi sverkhsmertnosit v Rossii [The alcohol catastrophe and the possibilities of public policy in overcoming extreme alcohol mortality in Russia],* 2nd ed. Moscow, URSS.

Rossow I (2001). Alcohol and homicide: cross-cultural comparison of the relationship in 14 European countries. *Addiction,* 96:77–92.

Rothman KJ, Greenland S, Lash TL (2008). *Modern Epidemiology,* 3rd ed. Philadelphia, PA, Lippincott Williams & Wilkins.

Schütze N et al. (2011). Alcohol attributable burden of incidence of cancer in eight European countries based on results from prospective cohort study. *British Medical Journal,* 342:d1584.

Shield K, Rehm J. Difficulties with telephone-based surveys on alcohol in high-income countries: the Canadian example. *International Journal of Methods in Psychiatric Research*, doi: 10.1002/mpr.1345.

Skog OJ (2001). Alcohol consumption and overall accident mortality in 14 European countries. *Addiction,* S35–S47.

Spode H (1993). *Die Macht der Trunkenheit: Kultur- und Sozialgeschichte des Alkohols in Deutschland Opladen.* Leverkusen, Germany, Verlag Leske & Budrich GmbH.

WHO (2004). *Global status report on alcohol and health.* Geneva, World Health Organization.

WHO (2011). *Global status report on alcohol and health.* Geneva, World Health Organization.

WHO (2012). Global Information System on Alcohol and Health (GISAH) [online database]. Geneva, World Health Organization (http://who.int/globalatlas/alcohol, accessed 23 February 2012).

Wittchen HU et al. (2011). The size and burden of mental disorders and other disorders of the brain in Europe 2010. *European Neuropsychopharmacology,* 21:655–679.

Zatonski W, Manczuk M, Sulkowska U (2008). In: *Closing the health gap in European Union.* Warsaw, Cancer Epidemiology and Prevention Division, The Maria Sklodowska-Curie Memorial Cancer Centre and Institute of Oncology.

Zatonski W et al. (2010). Liver cirrhosis mortality in Europe, with special attention to central and eastern Europe. *European Addiction Research,* 16:193–201.

Unrecorded and illicit alcohol

Dirk W Lachenmeier

Introduction

The EC report, *Alcohol in Europe. A public health perspective* (Anderson & Baumberg, 2006), considered unrecorded alcohol as a dimension of the economic and public health impact of alcohol in Europe. Based on Hvalkof & Anderson (1995), the report defined unrecorded alcohol consumption as "alcohol consumption which is not reflected in official statistics on alcohol consumption".

Although unrecorded consumption is by its nature difficult to measure, WHO figures (Rehm et al., 2004) show that illicit and cross-border consumptions seem to be highest in eastern Europe (particularly the Baltic countries, Bulgaria and Slovenia). Based on a tentative estimate of trends in unrecorded consumption, such consumption has been increasing since the mid-1970s in the Nordic countries and the United Kingdom while remaining stable elsewhere in the countries belonging to the EU before May 2004 (Leifman, 2001). No information on trends was available in the countries joining the EU in May 2004.

The amount of unrecorded consumption of alcohol in the EU is currently about 13% of all alcohol consumed, but with marked differences between the European countries (Table 1).

The following problems related to unrecorded and illicit alcohol currently occur in the EU:

- illegal production, tax fraud, counterfeiting and smuggling of alcoholic beverages leads to loss of tax income for governments, to a distortion of competition leading to loss of income for the honest trade, and to deception of the consumer if such products are sold as being legally produced;
- surrogate alcohol (alcohol not originally intended for human consumption) may additionally pose health risks due to toxic denaturants or additives (for example, in cosmetic alcohol);
- the large-scale marketing of illegal or surrogate alcohol may be interconnected with organized crime;
- cross-border shopping in the Nordic countries may undermine national alcohol policy (particularly if this occurs on a larger scale including (private) sale to others);
- home production of wine, beer and spirits may occur (depending on country, type of alcohol or annual production amount, this may be legal or illegal, registered or not registered);
- all these forms of unrecorded alcohol (except of cross-border shopping and registered home production) may pose a hazard for the consumer due to a lack of control by EU production hygiene regulations and of compliance with EU regulations regarding product quality and safety (for example, undetected methanol contents may lead to fatal poisoning).

Regarding health outcomes, no unique effects of unrecorded alcohol were pointed out other than an association with anomalously high rates of liver cirrhosis in Hungary, Romania and Slovenia.

It was speculated that aliphatic alcohol congeners (so-called higher alcohols) arising from homemade spirits increase the risk of liver cirrhosis (Szücs et al., 2005).

Regarding the economic impact, the major problem was thought to be smuggling and tax fraud. Such illegal trade occurs, for example, by diverting goods that are held in duty suspension (alcoholic beverages within the EU may move in duty suspension where the tax is only paid when and where the goods are released for consumption). The fraud occurs when the goods are illegally diverted from their (low-tax) claimed destination to a new (high-tax) one. While it is difficult to obtain reliable statistics on illicit trade, the European High Level Group on Fraud has estimated that €1.5 billion was lost to alcohol fraud in 1996. The level of governmental enforcement is obviously a factor affecting the level of smuggling and fraudulent activity.

As well as smuggling, there may be tax losses or shifts between countries via cross-border shopping, especially when there are large price differentials across small distances such as have occurred in the Nordic countries. Trends in legitimate cross-border shopping were on the rise as a result of the relaxation of travellers' allowances for intra-EU purchases.

Apart from the need for improved enforcement against smuggling, the report provided no policy options specific to the other types of unrecorded alcohol (such as home production). However, it was pointed out that further research would need unrecorded consumption to be measured, particularly in the countries joining the EU in May 2004.

Updated evidence

In 2009, the Regional Office (WHO Regional Office for Europe, 2009) provided an update on the effectiveness and cost–effectiveness of interventions to reduce alcohol-related harm (Table 5). The book considered unrecorded alcohol in more detail than did Anderson & Baumberg (2006), including a chapter dedicated to the reduction of the public health impact of unrecorded alcohol. First and foremost, the book provided an updated definition of unrecorded alcohol (see Box 2). Further details about definition and examples are provided in Lachenmeier, Gmel & Rehm (in press).

In order to combat smuggling, illegal trade and diversion fraud, which are believed to have increased in some EU member states, the EC and member states have taken some initiatives, including the adoption of a Commission Recommendation concerning warehouse-keepers, and the computerization of the movement and surveillance system of excisable products.

In settings with higher levels of unrecorded production and consumption, increasing the proportion of consumption that is taxed may represent a more effective pricing policy than a simple increase in excise tax, which may only encourage further illegal production, smuggling and cross-border shopping (WHO Regional Office for Europe, 2009). As no data on the full extent of smuggled alcohol are available, no evidence-based research about the effectiveness and cost–effectiveness of these measures is currently available.

While smuggled alcohol (especially from diversion fraud) will most likely be of similar quality to legally traded alcohol, the WHO Regional Office for Europe (2009) pointed out that surrogate and home-produced alcohol could be more detrimental to health due to contamination with substances added either as a denaturant (methanol) or flavouring (coumarin in cosmetic alcohol) or inadvertently introduced during home-production (ethyl carbamate or lead). The foremost problem from these may be methanol, which has led to several outbreaks of acute poisoning in the past (Lachenmeier, Rehm & Gmel, 2007). An effective policy measure to reduce methanol-

Table 5. An updated evidence base on unrecorded alcohol

Type of unrecorded alcohol	Policy option	Reference
All	Europe-wide tax stamps and mechanisms to track the movements of all alcohol products in the distribution chain, including effective enforcement of laws, should be introduced.	WHO Regional Office for Europe (2009); Babor et al. (2010)
All	In countries with high levels of unrecorded production and consumption, increasing the proportion of consumption that is taxed could be more effective than a simple increase in excise taxes.	Babor et al. (2010)
Cross-border trade	Lowering tax rates on alcohol to offset cross-border trade or an illicit market in alcohol can bring the risk of extra alcohol-related harm.	WHO Regional Office for Europe (2009)
Smuggled alcohol	Producers and retailers could commit themselves to sharing intelligence and knowledge of illegally traded and illicit alcohol.	WHO Regional Office for Europe (2009)
Surrogate alcohol	The use of methanol or methanol-containing products should be disallowed as denaturing agents.	WHO Regional Office for Europe (2009)
Surrogate alcohol	The use of substances with unfavourable toxic profile if consumed (such as polyhexamethyleneguanidine hydrochloride (PHMG) or coumarin) should be disallowed in consumer products.	Lachenmeier, Taylor & Rehm (2011)
Surrogate alcohol	Surrogate alcohols could be treated with bittering agents to avoid consumption.	WHO Regional Office for Europe (2009)
Medicinal alcohol	Rigorous controls should be introduced on the sale of medicinal alcohol and only small container sizes permitted.	WHO Regional Office for Europe (2009)
Home production	Financial incentives could be offered to the producers for registration and quality control.	Lachenmeier, Taylor & Rehm (2011)

Box 2. Definition of unrecorded alcohol

Unrecorded alcohol is:
- home-made;
- illegally produced; or
- smuggled alcohol products; as well as
- surrogate alcohol that is not officially intended for human consumption (mouthwash, perfumes and eau-de-colognes).

Source: WHO Regional Office for Europe, 2009.

---

attributable morbidity and mortality is to disallow the use of methanol (or methanol-containing wood alcohol) as a denaturing agent, as is the case in some EU countries (European Commission, 1993).

Recent research has shown that fears about the toxicity of unrecorded alcohol are mostly exaggerated (Rehm, Kanteres & Lachenmeier, 2010). For example, quantitative risk comparisons have shown that the potency of ethanol for liver toxicity is at least 5000-fold higher than that of ethyl carbamate (Lachenmeier, Kanteres & Rehm, 2011). Exposure to higher levels of alcohol from home-produced spirits also does not exceed toxicological thresholds and cannot explain the high rates of liver cirrhosis in Hungary, Romania and Slovenia mentioned above (Lachenmeier, Haupt & Schulz, 2008). Rather than by alcohol quality, the liver cirrhosis rates could be as well explained by a higher alcoholic strength of the unrecorded alcohol consumed, problematic drinking patterns, lower socioeconomic status and poor health status and the interaction effect of these factors (Rehm, Kanteres & Lachenmeier, 2010).

A large industry-financed study in the Russian Federation was also not able to find substantial differences in toxicity between home-produced and commercial spirits (Nuzhnyi, 2004). The exception may be the occurrence of PHMG, which was associated with an outbreak of acute cholestatic liver injury in the Russian Federation connected to the consumption of surrogate alcohol (Ostapenko et al., 2011). The alcohol that was consumed was a liquid for indoor disinfection containing PHMG as an antiseptic compound.

The evidence base on policy measures regarding unrecorded alcohol has recently been reviewed (Lachenmeier, Taylor & Rehm, 2011). Besides the policy options discussed by the Regional Office (WHO Regional Office for Europe, 2009) and Babor et al. (2010), the review article (Lachenmeier, Taylor & Rehm, 2011) provides a detailed discussion regarding small-scale artisanal home production of alcohol. On the basis of historic examples from western Europe, the authors concluded that incentive-based systems (intended to bring home production under state control) probably work better than prohibiting home production, which is difficult to enforce.

There are two EU-financed projects that deal with unrecorded alcohol (see Annex 4).

Influence of price policies on the informal market

The disadvantage of pricing policies is that the informal or illicit market for alcohol in some countries can complicate policy in this area by shifting consumption to unrecorded beverages (Babor et al., 2010). Thus, the measures discussed in this chapter are needed concomitantly in a comprehensive alcohol policy approach. The alcohol industry regularly lobbies against tax increases with clearly exaggerated fears about the public health impact of unrecorded alcohol (Lachenmeier & Rehm, 2009). There is also evidence that there is never a complete substitution between beverage types following price changes (Babor et al., 2010). Nevertheless, it must be mentioned that alcohol policy science provides comparably weak evidence as to the effectiveness of measures against unrecorded alcohol in general, and of measures against substitution when pricing and taxation are being adjusted in particular (Lachenmeier, Taylor & Rehm, 2011; Babor et al., 2010).

Conclusions for practice and policy

It was already known that the chemical composition of unrecorded alcohol is unlikely to pose a substantial health hazard beyond the effects of ethanol (WHO Regional Office for Europe, 2009; Lachenmeier et al., 2011), except in the rare cases (especially in the EU) of methanol poisoning (Lachenmeier, Rehm & Gmel, 2007) .

The current state of research shows that the surplus health hazards of unrecorded alcohol predominantly arise from: (i) a higher potential intake of ethanol compared to the same volume of commercial alcohol, because unrecorded alcohol is typically higher in alcoholic strength; (ii) a higher potential intake of ethanol, as unrecorded alcohol is cheaper than recorded alcohol; and (iii) anecdotal evidence that the patterns of drinking could be more detrimental for unrecorded than for recorded consumption.

Research gaps

The first step to address unrecorded alcohol is to provide better estimates of the size of the market and of measurement of the amount of consumption (Anderson & Baumberg, 2006).

As the policy measures largely depend on the type of unrecorded alcohol (for example, home production requires different measures to those needed for large-scale smuggling), insight into a country- or region-specific distribution of consumption between the categories of unrecorded alcohol is also required. Reliable consumption data over time are also required to provide adequate monitoring of the effectiveness of policy measures.

Conclusions

The following conclusions should be helpful for policy and practice.

- Unrecorded alcohol consumption is highest in eastern Europe, particularly the Baltic countries, Bulgaria and Slovenia.

- The major economic impact comes from losses due to smuggling and tax fraud. The level of illegal trade and smuggling predominantly depends on the level of governmental enforcement.

- Especially in settings with higher levels of unrecorded production and consumption, increasing the proportion of consumption that is taxed may represent a more effective pricing policy than simple increase in excise tax.

- The health effects and toxicity of unrecorded alcohol were found to be very similar to commercial alcohol, predominantly caused by ethanol itself. The major problem is certainly that unrecorded spirits are often sold at higher alcoholic strength (>45% vol) but for half the price of legal beverages, possibly leading to more detrimental patterns of drinking and overproportionate health hazards.

- Overall in the EU, the health risks from unrecorded alcohol are not much greater than would be true for an equivalent amount of recorded alcohol.

- To improve the knowledge base about unrecorded alcohol, better estimates of the size of the market and of the amount of consumption need to be provided. Insight into the distribution of consumption between the categories of unrecorded alcohol would be also required to provide a targeted country or region-specific policy response.

References

Anderson P, Baumberg B (2006). *Alcohol in Europe. A public health perspective*. London, Institute of Alcohol Studies (http://ec.europa.eu/health-eu/doc/alcoholineu_content_en.pdf, accessed 18 February 2012).

Babor TF et al. (2010). *Alcohol: no ordinary commodity. Research and public policy,* 2nd ed. Oxford, Oxford University Press.

European Commission (1993). Commission Regulation (EC) No 3199/93 of 22 November 1993 on the mutual recognition of procedures for the complete denaturing of alcohol for the purposes of exemption from excise duty. *Official Journal of the European Communities*, L288:12–15.

Hvalkof S, Anderson P (1995). *Terminology for alcohol policy.* Copenhagen, WHO Regional Office for Europe.

Lachenmeier DW, Gmel G, Rehm J (in press). Unrecorded alcohol consumption. In: Boyle P, Boffetta P, Lowenfels A, Burns H et al., eds. *Alcohol: science, policy and public health*. Oxford, Oxford University Press.

Lachenmeier DW, Haupt S, Schulz K (2008). Defining maximum levels of higher alcohols in alcoholic beverages and surrogate alcohol products. *Regulatory Toxicology and Pharmacology,* 50:313–321.

Lachenmeier DW, Kanteres F, Rehm J (2011). Epidemiology-based risk assessment using the benchmark dose/margin of exposure approach: the example of ethanol and liver cirrhosis. *International Journal of Epidemiology*, 40:210–218.

Lachenmeier DW, Leitz J, Schoeberl K et al. (2011b) Quality of illegally and informally produced alcohol in Europe: results from the AMPHORA project. *Adicciones*, 23:133–140.

Lachenmeier DW, Rehm J (2009). Unrecorded alcohol: A threat to public health? *Addiction*, 104: 875–877.

Lachenmeier DW, Rehm J, Gmel G (2007). Surrogate alcohol: what do we know and where do we go? *Alcoholism: Clinical and Experimental Research*, 31:1613–1624.

Lachenmeier DW, Taylor BJ, Rehm J (2011). Alcohol under the radar: do we have policy options regarding unrecorded alcohol? *International Journal of Drug Policy*, 22:153–160.

Leifman H (2001). Estimations of unrecorded alcohol consumption levels and trends in 14 European countries. *Nordisk Alkohol- & Narkotikatidskrift*; 18(English Suppl.):54–70.

Nuzhnyi V (2004). Chemical composition, toxic, and organoleptic properties of noncommercial alcohol samples. In: Haworth A, Simpson R, eds. *Moonshine markets. Issues in unrecorded alcohol beverage production and consumption.* New York, NY, Brunner-Routledge:177–199.

Ostapenko YN et al. (2011). Acute cholestatic liver injury caused by polyhexamethyleneguanidine hydrochloride admixed to ethyl alcohol. *Clinical Toxicology*, 40: 471–477.

Rehm J, Kanteres F, Lachenmeier DW (2010). Unrecorded consumption, quality of alcohol and health consequences. *Drug and Alcohol Review*, 29:426–436.

Rehm J et al. (2004). Alcohol use. In: Ezzati M, Lopez AD, Rodgers A, Murray CJL, eds. *Comparative quantification of health risks. Global and regional burden of disease attributable to selected major risk factors. Vol. 1.* Geneva, World Health Organization:959–1108.

Szücs S et al. (2005). Could the high level of cirrhosis in central and eastern Europe be due partly to the quality of alcohol consumed? An exploratory investigation. *Addiction*, 100:536–542.

WHO Regional Office for Europe (2009). *Evidence for the effectiveness and cost–effectiveness of interventions to reduce alcohol-related harm.* Copenhagen, WHO Regional Office for Europe (http://www.euro.who.int/__data/assets/pdf_file/0020/43319/E92823.pdf, accessed 12 February 2012).

Information and education

Peter Anderson

Introduction

In 2006, it was concluded that there was limited evidence for the effectiveness of public service announcements and public education campaigns (particularly those focusing on low-risk drinking guidelines), although media advocacy approaches could be important to gain public support for policy changes (Anderson & Baumberg, 2006). Likewise there was limited evidence for the impact of warning labels, although there was an argument for their use in relation to consumer protection and consumer rights. There were individual examples of the beneficial impact of school-based education, but systematic reviews and meta-analyses found that the majority of well-evaluated studies showed no impact, even in the short term. There was considerable experience of what might be best practice in school-based education programmes, but unconvincing evidence of their effectiveness. This is not to imply that education programmes should not be delivered, since all people do need to be informed about the use of alcohol and the harm done by it, but school-based education should not be seen as the only and simple answer to reduce the harm done by alcohol.

School-based information and education

Many systematic reviews have evaluated school-based education and concluded that classroom-based education is not effective in reducing alcohol-related harm (Foxcroft et al., 2003; Jones et al., 2007). Although there is evidence of positive effects arising from increased knowledge about alcohol and improved alcohol-related attitudes, there is no evidence for a sustained effect on behaviour. One systematic review of 14 systematic reviews identified 59 high-quality programmes, of which only 6 were able to demonstrate any evidence of effectiveness (Jones et al., 2007). Another systematic review of the impact of universal school-based prevention programmes for alcohol reported in 2011 found 53 trials (Foxcroft & Tsertsvadze, 2011a). However, estimating the overall impact was hampered by poor reporting quality in almost all the trials. Of the 11 trials that evaluated alcohol-specific interventions, 5 found no effect and 6 found some evidence of effect in some outcome measures. Of the 39 trials that evaluated generic interventions, 25 found no effect and 14 found some evidence of effect in some outcome measures. The most commonly observed positive effects across programmes were for drunkenness and binge-drinking. Unfortunately, it was not possible to identify any characteristics that distinguished trials with positive results from those with no effects. It is interesting to note that one of the series of reviews that did find a positive outcome (Tobler et al., 2000) was based on inappropriate analyses which, on proper analysis, found no effect (McCambridge, 2007).

It has been suggested that parenting programmes might have more promise but, even here, mixed effects have been found. For example, a systematic review of 14 parenting programmes found reductions in alcohol use in only 6 programmes (Petrie, Bunn & Byrne, 2007). Another systematic review of the impact of family-based prevention programmes for alcohol reported in 2011 found 12 studies reporting 9 trials (not 12 trials as reported in the review) (Foxcroft & Tsertsvadze, 2011b). Three of the nine trials found no effect. In the remaining six trials, there was evidence for effect, although this was not consistent across all outcome measures and time periods.

It has also been suggested that social marketing programmes might have more promise but, even here, mixed effects have been found. A systematic review of 15 social marketing programmes found 8 out of 13 studies showing some significant effects on alcohol use in the short term (up to 12 months), 4 out of 7 studies showing some effect at 1–2 years, and 2 out of 4 studies showing some effect over 2 years (Stead et al., 2007).

A systematic review of the impact of multicomponent prevention programmes for alcohol reported in 2011 found 20 trials (Foxcroft & Tsertsvadze, 2011c). In general, the scientific quality and reporting of the trials was poor. Of the 20 trials, 8 found no effect. There was some evidence for some positive outcomes in the remaining 12, but in only 4 studies was the effect consistent across the range of outcome measures used. From this review, it cannot be reliably concluded that multicomponent interventions for the prevention of alcohol-related harm in young people is effective.

A systematic review of preventive interventions addressing under-age drinking identified 25 reviews and over 400 interventions. The evidence for 127 of these was reviewed and only 12 were found to have promising evidence on alcohol outcomes (Spoth, Greenberg & Turrisi, 2008). The promising interventions were mixed, and it was not possible to identify any clear group or category of programme that showed promise.

While education primarily aims to affect behaviour through influencing attitudes, there is some evidence to suggest that in fact attitudes are influenced by behaviour, thus raising the question of whether interventions should focus on attitudes or behaviour. Research in adolescent smoking has found that attitudes towards smoking were neither consistent nor strong predictors of smoking behaviour over time (de Leeuw et al., 2008). The same study found that in fact, past smoking was related to attitudes indicating that adolescents adapted their attitudes to match their behaviour. It also suggested that other factors play important roles in beginning and continuing to smoke, such as favourable social images and peers who smoke.

Public education campaigns

In general, public information campaigns have been found to be ineffective in reducing alcohol-related harm (Babor et al., 2010). Exceptions are mass media campaigns to reduce drinking and driving which, when implemented in the presence of strong drinking and driving countermeasures, can have an impact (Elder et al., 2004). Counter-advertising, a variant of public information campaigns which provides information about a product, its effects and the industry that promotes it in order to decrease its appeal and use, has inconclusive effects (Babor et al., 2010).

Campaigns based on drinking guidelines

While campaigns based on drinking guidelines have been used in some countries, there have been no rigorous evaluations as to whether publicizing such guidelines has any impact on alcohol-related harm (Babor et al., 2010). In 2009, the Australian National Health and Medical Research Council released a revision of Australia's official low-risk alcohol guidelines, specifying low-risk consumption levels for both short- and long-term consumption. Large general population surveys run in 2007 and 2010 provided before and after measures of respondents' estimates of low-risk drinking levels (Livingstone, 2012). In the 2010 survey, fewer than 5% of respondents estimated low-risk drinking levels that matched those in the 2009 guidelines. Generally speaking, younger respondents and heavier drinkers provided higher estimates of low-risk drinking thresholds. There was little change in the estimates between 2007 and 2010.

Social responsibility messages

There is evidence that social responsibility messages from alcohol manufacturers or retailers, whether stand-alone or when added to product advertisements, benefit the reputation of the sponsor more than they do public health. For example, a study that assessed the impact of adding drink–driving messages to bar advertisements showed that inclusion of the message had positive effects on the perception of the advertiser in terms of concern about the safety of bar customers, but did not affect the attitudes or intentions variables (Christie, 2001). Similarly, another study found the message in alcohol industry social responsibility spots to be ambiguous, especially for the group aged 16–18 years, but that the source of the message (the alcohol company) was favourably perceived. Two thirds of the sample perceived the spots to be fairly or very similar to beer commercials, with over two thirds agreeing that the spots suggested that beer drinking was fun (Smith, Atkin & Roznowski, 2006). A recent review indicated that ambiguity and inconsistency in the use of the "responsible drinking" concept in alcohol advertising and public health commentary is widespread and conducive to misunderstanding (Barry & Goodson, 2010).

Consumer labelling and warning messages

In France, since 2007 a health warning has been placed on alcoholic drinks packaging in order to promote abstinence during pregnancy, supported by a press campaign and extensive media coverage. Two telephone surveys were conducted in 2004 and 2007 among two independent representative quota samples of the French population aged 15 years and over (approximately 1000 people interviewed in each survey) (Guillemont & Leon, 2008). It was found that the recommendation that pregnant women should not drink alcohol was better known after the introduction of the health warning (87% of the respondents) than before (82%) ($p<0.001$). After the introduction of the label, 30% thought that the risk for the fetus started after the first glass compared with 25% in 2004 ($p<0.01$). These rather modest results contrast with evidence from tobacco, where there is evidence of impact although it may reflect the nature of the warning labels, since it seems that the introduction of more graphic and larger warnings for cigarettes, with rotating messages, has affected behaviour (Borland et al., 2009). Nevertheless, warning labels are important in helping to establish a social understanding that alcohol is a special and hazardous commodity (Wilkinson & Room, 2009).

What to do about education and information

When looking at education alone, the lack of evidence for effectiveness could lead to policy-makers considering withdrawing funds from education programmes altogether. This would involve several risks, including: losing the importance of education for society in improving individual capital; losing an important means of gaining awareness of and support for other control measures; and leaving a gap which may be filled by industry-backed programmes. Many education programmes focus on young people, and there is evidence that young adults and adults are often overlooked; it is easier for young people to see such programmes as hypocritical when adults are left alone. Young adults and adults often serve as drinking role models for young people and also support easy access to alcohol, which is associated with increased drinking in all age groups, and are therefore an important target audience (Giesbrecht, 2007). The conceptual shift from influencing attitudes to affecting behaviour to looking at the influence of behaviour on attitudes is important to consider, especially among young people. It may be more effective to focus education/information activities on policy-makers and the general public as a means to raise awareness of the burden of alcohol-related harm and the benefits of effective measures to reduce this harm. Interventions could be reframed to encourage and support consumer advocacy by providing information on how the public can influence alcohol policy.

Conclusions

The following conclusions should be helpful for policy and practice.

- There is extensive evidence that school-based information and education programmes do not consistently lead to sustained changes in behaviour.

- Although they show some promise, there is no consistent evidence to demonstrate that parenting programmes and social marketing programmes lead to sustained changes in behaviour.

- Although poorly researched, there is no consistent evidence that public education campaigns lead to sustained changes in behaviour.

- There are no rigorous evaluations to demonstrate whether or not campaigns based on drinking guidelines lead to sustained changes in behaviour.

- Although there is limited research, there is some evidence that social responsibility campaigns by the alcohol industry can be counterproductive due to ambiguity and mixed messages.

- There is some evidence to show that consumer labelling and warning messages do not lead to sustained changes in behaviour.

Information and education on the risks from alcohol and how to reduce them is needed for an educated population and for the development of individual capital, although as an isolated policy measure it will not reduce alcohol-related harm. Education policy could benefit from incorporating a conceptual shift from influencing attitudes to affect behaviour to looking at the influence of behaviour on attitudes. Education and information activities could be reframed to encourage and support consumer advocacy by providing information on how the public can influence alcohol policy.

References

Anderson P, Baumberg B (2006). *Alcohol in Europe. A public health perspective*. London, Institute of Alcohol Studies (http://ec.europa.eu/health-eu/doc/alcoholineu_content_en.pdf, accessed 18 February 2012).

Babor TF et al. (2010). *Alcohol: no ordinary commodity. Research and public policy,* 2nd ed. Oxford, Oxford University Press.

Barry A, Goodson P (2010). Use (and misuse) of the responsible drinking message in public health and alcohol advertising: a review. *Health Education & Behavior*, 37(2):288–303.

Borland R et al. (2009). How reactions to cigarette packet health warnings influence quitting: findings from the ITC Four-Country survey. *Addiction,* 104:669–675.

Christie J et al. (2001). The effects of bar-sponsored alcohol beverage promotions across binge and nonbinge drinkers. *Journal of Public Policy & Marketing,* 20(2):240–253.

de Leeuw RNH et al. (2008). Do smoking attitudes predict behaviour? A longitudinal study on the bi-directional relations between adolescents' smoking attitudes and behaviours. *Addiction,* 103(10):1713–1721.

Elder RW et al. (2004). Effectiveness of mass media campaigns for reducing drinking and driving and alcohol-involved crashes: a systematic review. *American Journal of Preventive Medicine,* 27:57–65.

Foxcroft DR et al. (2003). Longer-term primary prevention for alcohol misuse in young people: a systematic review. *Addiction,* 98:397–411.

Foxcroft DR, Tsertsvadze A (2011a). Universal school-based prevention programs for alcohol misuse in young people. *Cochrane Database of Systematic Reviews,* (5):CD009113.

Foxcroft DR, Tsertsvadze A (2011b). Universal family-based prevention programs for alcohol misuse in young people. *Cochrane Database of Systematic Reviews*, (9):CD009308.

Foxcroft DR, Tsertsvadze A (2011c). Universal multicomponent prevention programs for alcohol misuse in young people. *Cochrane Database of Systematic Reviews,* (9):CD009307.

Giesbrecht N (2007). Reducing alcohol-related damage in populations: rethinking the roles of education and persuasion interventions. *Addiction,* 102:1345–1349.

Guillemont J, Léon C (2008). Alcool et grossesse: connaissances du grand public en 2007 et évolutions en trois ans. *Évolutions,* 15 (http://www.inpes.sante.fr/CFESBases/catalogue/pdf/ 1117.pdf, accessed 8 February 2012).

Jones L et al. (2007). *A review of the effectiveness and cost effectiveness of interventions delivered in primary and secondary schools to prevent and/or reduce alcohol use by young people under 18 years old.* London, National Institute for Health and Clinical Excellence (http://www.nice.org.uk/nicemedia/pdf/AlcoholSchoolsConsReview.pdf, accessed 8 February 2012).

Livingston M (2012). Perceptions of low-risk drinking levels among Australians during a period of change in the official drinking guidelines. *Drug and Alcohol Review*, 10.1111/j.1465-3362.2011.00414.x.

McCambridge J (2007). A case study of publication bias in an influential series of reviews of drug education. *Drug and Alcohol Review,* 26:463–468.

Petrie J, Bunn F, Byrne G (2007). Parenting programmes for preventing tobacco, alcohol and drug misuse in children <18 years: a systematic review. *Health Education Research,* 22(2):177–191.

Smith SW, Atkin CK, Roznowski J (2006). Are "Drink Responsibly" alcohol campaigns strategically ambiguous? *Health Communication,* 20(1):1–11.

Spoth R, Greenberg M, Turrisi R (2008). Preventive interventions addressing underage drinking: state of the evidence and steps toward public health impact. *Pediatrics,* 121:S311–S336.

Stead M, Gordon R, Angus K (2007). A systematic review of social marketing effectiveness. *Health Education*, 107(2):126–191.

Tobler N et al. (2000). School-based adolescent drug prevention programs: 1998 meta-analysis. *Journal of Primary Prevention,* 20:275–336.

Wilkinson C, Room R (2009). Informational and warning labels on alcohol containers, sales, places and advertisements: experience internationally and evidence on effects. *Drug and Alcohol Review*, 28(4):341–461.

Health sector responses

Eileen Kaner

Introduction

Up to 2006, a large amount of high-quality evidence had accumulated to support the effectiveness of health sector interventions in reducing alcohol-related harm (Anderson & Baumberg, 2006; Miller & Wilbourne, 2002). The largest and most robust body of evidence related to preventive interventions, particularly brief alcohol interventions. In 2006, there were 14 systematic reviews (with or without meta-analyses) which assessed the impact of brief interventions on reducing alcohol consumption, some of which also considered their impact on ameliorating alcohol-related problems. The most comprehensive review included 56 controlled trials (Moyer et al., 2002) and encompassed a wide range of delivery settings and patients who were either not aware of their alcohol-related risk or harm (non-treatment-seekers) or aware and seeking help for problems (treatment-seekers). Thirty-four trials focused on non-treatment-seekers and reported that brief interventions produced small to medium aggregate effect sizes (range 0.14 to 0.67) over a range of time points. For the 20 trials that focused on treatment-seekers, the overall brief intervention effect size was not significantly different from zero (range -0.02 to 0.4). The modal follow-up time was 1 year and there was mixed evidence of longer-term effects, with positive outcomes reported at 4 years in the United States (Fleming et al., 2002) but not at 10 years in Australia (Wutzke et al., 2002). There was also evidence that brief intervention could reduce mortality (Cuijpers, Riper & Lemmers 2004) and other alcohol-related problems (Moyer et al., 2002; Richmond et al., 1995). The number needed to treat was between 8 and 12 for hazardous and harmful drinkers (Ballesteros et al., 2004). This is the number of at-risk drinkers who needed to be offered brief interventions for one to show benefit in terms of reduced drinking levels or fewer alcohol-related problems.

Most of this brief intervention research was based in primary care, where the evidence of a positive impact was strongest (Ballesteros et al., 2004; Bertholet et al., 2005; Whitlock et al., 2004). WHO's CHOosing Interventions that are Cost Effective (CHOICE) model estimated that delivery of primary care-based brief interventions to 25% of the at-risk population throughout Europe could prevent around 408 000 years of disability and premature death at an estimated cost of €740 million each year (Chisholm et al., 2004). Just one systematic review focused on emergency care, and this reported 27% to 65% reductions in a range of trauma and injury measures (Dinh-Zarr et al., 1999). Less evidence was available for other settings but individual studies showed a beneficial impact of brief interventions targeting pregnant women (Handmaker, Miller & Manicke, 1999; Handmaker et al., 2006). There was also evidence that home-visit interventions could reduce harmful alcohol use in pregnancy (Grant et al., 2005). Regarding occupational health settings, there was evidence that brief interventions could reduce alcohol consumption in those experiencing the intervention (Richmond et al., 2000) and that a brief eight- hour training programme reduced problem drinking from 20% to 11% and linked absenteeism from 16% to 6% (Bennett et al., 2004).

Regarding alcohol treatment, the strongest evidence was reported for behavioural skill training and pharmacotherapy interventions (Miller & Wilbourne, 2002). Areas with less impact were 12-step facilitation, group psychotherapy, educational lectures and films, mandatory attendance at Alcoholics Anonymous meetings and general alcoholism counselling.

Recent evidence

A great deal of evidence has emerged since 2006 (WHO, 2009; Babor et al., 2010; Babor et al., in press), particularly relating to brief interventions in non-treatment-seekers (Table 6). In the last five years, three further systematic reviews have focused on primary care (Kaner et al., 2007; Littlejohn, 2006; Saitz, 2010), two on emergency care (Havard, Shakeshaft & Sanson-Fisher, 2008; Nilsen et al., 2008), one on general hospital settings (McQueen et al., 2011) and two on obstetric or antenatal care (Doggett, Burrett & Osborne, 2009; Stade et al., 2009). Most reviews included delivery of brief interventions by doctors, but a recent review focused on non-physician delivery (Sullivan et al., 2011). Two further systematic reviews specifically considered economic outcomes (Bray et al., 2011) and impact on co-morbid conditions (Kaner, Brown & Jackson, 2011). Other relevant systematic reviews considered motivational interviewing across some behaviour patterns (Lundahl et al., 2010) and brief interventions beyond the health sector to educational and/or community settings (Peltzer, 2009; Tripodi et al., 2010). Across this wide body of work, it has been reported that brief interventions have consistently reduced the quantity, frequency or intensity of drinking (Kaner et al., 2007). The beneficial effects of brief interventions continued to be particularly strong in primary care (Kaner et al., 2007). Brief intervention outcomes in emergency care, general hospital settings and obstetric or antenatal care were more equivocal, with both positive and null findings. An enduring theme was that brief interventions relating to alcohol have a greater impact on non-treatment-seeking patients compared to treatment-seekers in specialist settings (Kaner, Brown & Jackson, 2011). Delivery by a range of practitioners has beneficial effects, although the size of these effects was greater when doctors were the deliverers (Sullivan et al., 2011). Moreover, brief interventions have been found to reduce overall health costs but not subsequent inpatient or outpatient utilization of health services (Bray et al., 2011). Nevertheless, a recent comprehensive overview of systematic reviews in this area, conducted for the National Institute for Health and Clinical Excellence in England, concluded that screening together with brief interventions for alcohol was a highly cost-effective strategy for health sector organizations (Latimer et al., 2010).

Most of the brief intervention evidence base has focused on adults rather than young or elderly people. In addition, a recent WHO review concluded that this evidence base has limited applicability to low- and middle-income countries (Babor et al., in press). One innovation in this field which may help to extend the reach of brief interventions is the development of computerized or web-based approaches (e-interventions). A key feature of these e-interventions is that they may help to target younger people who tend not to present to health settings, and they may be used in contexts where health services are not fully developed. Nine recent systematic reviews have considered e-interventions (Bewick et al., 2008; Carey et al., 2007; Carey et al., 2009; Elliott, Carey & Bolles, 2008; Khadjesari et al., 2010; Moreira, Smith & Foxcroft, 2009; Riper et al., 2009; Rooke et al., 2010; White et al., 2010) and reported that they generally produce beneficial outcomes compared to controls who receive no interventions but rarely compared to other active interventions (Carey et al., 2009). Thus directly delivered, individually focused brief interventions are likely to yield more positive effects compared to indirectly delivered e-interventions. The latter do, however, have a promising reach into groups that are hard to access and have a relatively low cost once the initial intervention development work is completed.

An enduring finding from the brief intervention literature is that there is little evidence to suggest that longer or more intensive input provides additional benefit over shorter, simpler input (Kaner et al., 2007). So while personal contact may be important, the length, complexity and intensity of the intervention are likely to be less so. Moreover, two recent systematic reviews focused on the

Table 6. Systematic reviews since 2006 focused on brief interventions in the health sector

First author, year	Setting	No. of trials	Conclusions
Bernstein, 2010	Health	38	Meta-analysis of 16 trials found consistent drinking reductions in control groups (effect size 0.37).
Bewick, 2008	E-intervention	5	Evidence on the effectiveness of e-input was inconsistent. Web-based input was generally well received.
Bray, 2011	Health	29	Meta-analysis of 11 trials found no significant effect on outpatient or inpatient health care use.
Carey, 2007	Colleges	62	Face-to-face input of motivational interviewing and personalized normative feedback produce greater reductions than no-input controls.
Carey, 2009	E-intervention; colleges	35	E-intervention was beneficial compared to assessment-only controls but not compared to active comparators.
Doggett, 2009	Obstetric care	6	There was insufficient evidence to recommend routine home visits for women with alcohol/drug problems.
Elliot, 2008	E-intervention; colleges	17	E- input rarely produced greater effects than alternative alcohol risk reduction interventions.
Havard, 2008	Emergency care	10	Meta-analyses of direct and e-interventions showed that they did not significantly reduce consumption but that they reduced the odds of injury (odds ratio (OR): 0.59; 95% confidence interval (CI): 0.42–0.84).
Jenkins, 2009	Health and educational	22	There was a general but inconsistent trend for reduced drinking in control groups, and the effect was greater in anglophone countries.
Kaner, 2007	Primary care	29	Meta-analysis of 29 trials found significantly reduced consumption, particularly in men. Longer interventions had little additional benefit.
Kaner, 2011	Health	14	The review focused on co-morbidities and found positive outcomes for substance use and physical health (3 trials) but not substance use and mental health (8 trials) or dual substance use (3 trials).
Khadjesari, 2010	E-intervention; colleges	24	Meta-analysis of 19 trials found computer-input more effective than no-input controls. Few studies compared e-input with active comparator groups.
Lundahl, 2010	Health and social care	119	Meta-analysis of 68 alcohol trials found that motivational interviewing produced a significant impact compared to weak comparators (effect size 0.28) but not compared to other active treatments (effect size 0.09).
McQueen, 2011	Hospital settings	14	Meta-analysis of four trials found beneficial but time-limited effects of brief interventions with hospital inpatients.
Moreira, 2009	E-intervention; colleges	22	Web and individually focused feedback gave a short-term positive effect compared to controls but not when compared to each other. There were null effects for mail or group feedback and social norms marketing campaigns.
Nilsen, 2008	Emergency care	14	Most trials found positive effects on one or more outcomes. More intensive brief interventions yielded better effects. Five trials had null effects against active treatments.
Peltzer, 2009	Health, school, community	7	A small number of studies found a positive health sector impact. Community-setting outcomes were promising but brief interventions were usually combined with HIV counselling.
Riper, 2009	E-intervention; community	14	Single-session personalized-feedback had positive but modest effects. Eight internet trials had a broad reach.
Rooke, 2010	E-intervention; colleges	34	In 28 alcohol trials, e-interventions reduced alcohol use (effect size 0.22) with low cost.
Saitz, 2010	Primary care	16	There was a positive impact on unhealthy alcohol use, but not for patients with very heavy use or dependence.
Stade, 2009	Antenatal care	4	No meta-analysis was made and no significance was reported between group differences for most outcomes. There was little impact on health.
Sullivan, 2011	Health	13	A meta-analysis of six trials found a positive impact of non-physician input but the effect (1.7 fewer drinks per week) was greater when physicians made the input (2.7 fewer drinks per week).

First author, year	Setting	No. of trials	Conclusions
Tripodi, 2010	Health, social, educational	16	Psychosocial inputs were effective at reducing alcohol use (effect size -0.61). Individual inputs had a larger effect (-0.75) compared to family inputs (-0.46).
Vasilaki, 2006	Health, social, educational	22	A meta-analysis of 15 trials found a significant small impact compared to controls where there was no input (effect size 0.18) and a greater impact compared to active treatment (effect size 0.43).
White, 2010	E-intervention; workplaces, colleges	17	A meta-analysis of 8 trials found that online input could be effective but there was a wide range of effect sizes (0.02–0.88) owing to heterogeneity.

control groups in brief intervention trials (Bernstein, Bernstein & Heeren 2010; Jenkins, McAlaney & McCambridge, 2009) and reported consistently reduced drinking. Thus it has been suggested that screening or assessment reactivity may be important elements of positive brief intervention effects (McCambridge & Day, 207; Kypri et al., 2007).

Despite considerable efforts over the years to persuade practitioners to deliver brief interventions in practice, most have yet to do so. A systematic review of 12 studies found that a combination of educational and office support could increase short-term delivery of brief interventions in primary care from 32% to 45% (Anderson et al., 2004). Nevertheless, there continue to be challenges in implementing brief interventions in the health sector. A recent survey in England (Wilson et al., 2011) reported that while practitioners' attitudes have improved over the last decade (Kaner et al., 1999), this has not been matched by actual practice. Despite some progress in disseminating the supporting evidence base (Kaner, 2010) and in developing national guidance on brief interventions (NICE, 2010), a lack of time and reimbursement remain enduring obstacles for this work. Thus there is a need to encourage national and local policy-makers to find ways of incentivising and embedding this work in busy practice settings (McCormick, 2010).

One review bridged the divide between prevention and treatment by considering brief interventions in hospitalized patients (McQueen et al., 2011). While 14 randomized controlled trials were identified, primarily from the United Kingdom and United States, a varying number contributed to the meta-analyses of the various outcome measures (range 1–7 trials). The primary meta-analysis included four trials and found that patients receiving brief interventions showed greater reductions in alcohol consumption compared to controls at six months (mean difference: 69 g; 95% CI: -128 – -10) but not at one year. There were also significantly fewer deaths following brief interventions at six months (relative risk: 0.42; 95% CI: 0.19–0.94) and one year (relative risk: 0.60; 95% CI: 0.40–0.91). Thus, although a previous review had reported null effects from brief interventions in hospitalized patients, this updated review revised its conclusion to beneficial but time-limited effects. Nevertheless, it is not clear how many participants in the trial were alcohol treatment-seekers (aware of their alcohol problems before hospitalization) or non-treatment-seekers who became aware of their alcohol problem following hospitalization.

Four recent high-quality systematic reviews and meta-analyses have looked at specialist alcohol treatment, of which two focused on psychosocial counselling (Magill & Ray, 2009; Smedslund et al., 2011) and two focused on pharmacological treatment (Rösner et al., 2010a; Rösner et al., 2010b).

To date, 53 controlled trials have considered the impact of cognitive behavioural therapy (CBT) on substance use and 23 specifically on alcohol use (Magill & Ray, 2009). A small but clinically significant effect of CBT was reported, although its impact reduced over time from six months after the initial input (Magill & Ray, 2009). A large effect size was found for CBT compared to no treatment ($g=0.79$, $p <.005$; $n=6$), although a smaller effect was found for other comparison conditions (such as usual care or another active treatment). CBT combined with other psychosocial treatment showed a larger effect size ($g=0.30$, $p <.005$; $n=19$) than CBT combined with pharmacological treatment ($g=0.20$, $p <.005$; $n =13$) or CBT alone ($g=0.17$, $p <.05$; $n=21$). Regarding motivational interviewing approaches, 59 trials have focused on its impact on substance use and 29 trials on alcohol abuse or dependence (Smedslund et al., 2011). Compared to controls who received no treatment, motivational interviewing showed a significant impact in reducing substance use which was greatest soon after intervention (standardized mean difference: 0.79; 95% CI: 0.48–1.09) and reduced over time. For longer-term follow-up (12 months or longer), the effect was not significant (standardized mean difference: 0.06; 95% CI: -0.16–0.28). Motivational interviewing rarely produced significant benefits when compared to other active treatments.

Two key pharmacological therapies used to promote abstinence or reduced consumption in problem drinkers are acamprosate (a glutamate antagonist) and naltrexone (an opioid antagonist). In 2010, 2 systematic reviews identified 24 acamprosate trials (Rösner et al., 2010a) and 50 naltrexone trials (Rösner et al., 2010b). Compared to placebos, acamprosate significantly reduced the risk of drinking (relative risk: 0.86; 95% CI: 0.81–0.91) and the cumulative duration of abstinence reported by trial participants (mean difference: 10.94; 95% CI: 5.08–16.81) with minimal side-effects (Rösner et al., 2010a). Naltrexone reduced the risk of heavy drinking compared to a placebo group (relative risk: 0.83; 95% CI: 0.76–0.90) and significantly decreased the number of drinking days by about 4% (mean difference: -3.89; 95% CI: -5.75–-2.04). Positive effects were also demonstrated for some secondary outcomes including heavy drinking days, total alcohol consumption and gamma-glutamyltransferase (Rösner et al., 2010b). However, naltrexone gave side effects of mainly gastrointestinal problems and sedative effects (Rösner et al., 2010b).

In summary, there is a large literature on treatment which has emerged over recent years. These high-quality reviews have concluded that psychosocial counselling interventions generally produce beneficial but time-limited effects for patients and that pharmacological agents can be used to help achieve alcohol abstinence and other treatment outcomes in a safe and effective way. The precise combination of counselling and pharmacotherapy to use is less clear and must depend on the severity of the problem, the goals of treatment and the patient's preferences regarding possible side-effects.

Since 2006, the EU has increasingly supported projects aimed at promoting health sector responses to help reduce alcohol-related problems (see Annex 4).

Conclusions for policy and practice

There is a large and robust evidence base to support the effectiveness and cost–effectiveness of health sector responses in preventing and treating alcohol-related problems in EU member countries. The largest evidence base relates to preventive interventions, particularly the use of brief alcohol interventions with hazardous and harmful drinkers who are not seeking treatment, generally because they are unaware of their alcohol-related risk or harm. There have, however, been challenges in achieving wide-scale and or sustained implementation of brief interventions by practitioners. A range of EU projects have developed standardized tools to support the delivery of brief interventions and have identified strategies to help promote the uptake of these interventions in routine health care. Further support for the implementation of brief alcohol interventions in the health sector is likely to require clear prioritization of this issue in national public health strategies and incentives for this preventive work to be undertaken work by general practitioners, who often place more focus on treatment and care. Specialist practitioners have a range of therapies that can be used to help problem drinkers who are seeking treatment. A minority of problem drinkers tend, however, to present to services for this input. Improved screening and case detection approaches in primary care may help to address this problem. Finally, better integration of prevention and treatment services would also help to ensure that problem drinkers are fully supported by the health sector.

References

Anderson P, Baumberg B (2006). *Alcohol in Europe. A public health perspective*. London, Institute of Alcohol Studies (http://ec.europa.eu/health-eu/doc/alcoholineu_content_en.pdf, accessed 18 February 2012).

Anderson P et al. (2004). Engaging general practitioners in the management of alcohol problems: results of a meta-analysis. *Journal of Studies on Alcohol*, 65(2):191–199.

Babor TF et al. (2010). *Alcohol: no ordinary commodity – research and public policy*, 2nd ed. Oxford, Oxford University Press.

Babor T et al. (in press). *Rapid review of current evidence for health promotion actions for hazardous and harmful alcohol use, with specific reference to low- and middle-income countries: WHO mainstreaming health promotion project*. Geneva, World Health Organization.

Ballesteros JA et al. (2004). Efficacy of brief interventions for hazardous drinkers in primary care: systematic review and meta-analysis. *Alcoholism: Clinical and Experimental Research*, 28(4):608–618.

Bennett J et al. (2004). Team awareness, problem drinking, and drinking climate: workplace social health promotion in a policy context. *American Journal of Health Promotion*, 19(2):103–113.

Bernstein J, Bernstein E, Heeren T (2010). Mechanisms of change in control group drinking in clinical trials of brief alcohol intervention: implications for bias towards the null. *Drug and Alcohol Review*, 29:498–507.

Bertholet N et al. (2005). Brief alcohol intervention in primary care: systematic review and meta-analysis. *Archives of Internal Medicine*, 165:986–995.

Bewick BM et al. (2008). The effectiveness of web-based interventions designed to decrease alcohol consumption – a systematic review. *Preventive Medicine*, 47(1):17–26.

Bray JW, Cowell A, Hinde J (2011). A systematic review and meta-analysis of health care utilization outcomes in alcohol screening and brief intervention trials. *Medical Care*, 49:287–294.

Carey K, Scott-Sheldon L, Carey M (2007). Individual-level interventions to reduce college student drinking: a meta-analytic review. *Addictive Behaviors*, 32:2469–2494.

Carey K et al. (2009). Computer-delivered interventions to reduce college student drinking: a meta-analysis. *Addiction*, 104:1807–1819.

Chisholm D et al. (2004). Reducing the global burden of hazardous alcohol use: a comparative cost–effectiveness analysis. *Journal of Studies on Alcohol*, 65:782–793.

Cuijpers P, Riper H, Lemmers L (2004). The effects on mortality of brief interventions for problem drinking: a meta-analysis. *Addiction*, 99(7):839–845.

Dinh-Zarr T et al. (1999). Preventing injuries through intervention for problem drinking: a systematic review of randomized controlled trials. *Alcohol and Alcoholism*, 34(4): 609–621.

Doggett C, Burrett S, Osborne D (2009). Home visits during pregnancy and after birth for women with an alcohol or drug problem. *Cochrane Database of Systematic Reviews*, (4):CD004456.

Elliott JC, Carey KB, Bolles JR (2008). Computer based interventions for college drinking: a qualitative review. *Addictive Behaviours*, 33(8):994–1005.

Fleming MF et al. (2002). Brief physician advice for problem drinkers: long-term efficacy and benefit-cost analysis. *Alcoholism: Clinical and Experimental Research*, 26(1):36–43.

Grant T et al. (2005). Preventing alcohol and drug exposed births in Washington State: intervention findings from three parent-child assistance program sites. *American Journal of Drug and Alcohol Abuse*, 31(3):471–490.

Handmaker NS, Miller WR, Manicke M (1999). Findings of a pilot study of motivational interviewing with pregnant drinkers. *Journal of Studies on Alcohol*, 60:285–287.

Handmaker NS et al. (2006). Impact of alcohol exposure after pregnancy recognition on ultrasonographic fetal growth measures. *Alcoholism: Clinical and Experimental Research*, 30(5):892–898.

Havard A, Shakeshaft A, Sanson-Fisher R (2008). Systematic review and meta-analyses of strategies targeting alcohol problems in emergency departments: interventions reduce alcohol-related injuries. *Addiction*, 103:368–376.

Jenkins RJ, McAlaney J, McCambridge J (2009). Change over time in alcohol consumption in control groups in brief intervention studies: systematic review and meta-regression study. *Drug and Alcohol Dependence*, 100(1–2):107–114.

Kaner E (2010). Brief alcohol intervention: time for translational research. *Addiction*, 105:960–961.

Kaner EFS et al. (2007). Effectiveness of brief alcohol interventions in primary care populations. *Cochrane Database of Systematic Reviews*, (2):CD004148.

Kaner EFS, Brown N, Jackson K (2011). A systematic review of the impact of brief interventions on substance use and co-morbid physical and mental health conditions. *Mental Health and Substance Use*, 4(1):38–61.

Kaner EFS et al. (1999). Intervention for excessive alcohol consumption in primary health care: attitudes and practices of English general practitioners. *Alcohol and Alcoholism*, 34(4):559–566.

Khadjesari Z et al. (2010). Can stand-alone computer-based interventions reduce alcohol consumption? A systematic review. *Addiction*, 106:267–282.

Kypri K et al. (2007). Assessment may conceal therapeutic benefit: findings from a randomized controlled trial for hazardous drinking. *Addiction*, 102:62–70.

Latimer N et al. (2010). *Prevention and early identification of alcohol use disorders in adults and young people: screening and brief interventions, cost effectiveness review*. Sheffield, University of Sheffield, School of Health and Related Research (ScHARR) Public Health Collaborating Centre.

Littlejohn C (2006). Does socio-economic status influence the acceptability of, attendance for, and outcome of, screening and brief interventions for alcohol misuse: a review. *Alcohol and Alcoholism*, 41(5):540–545.

Lundahl B et al. (2010). A meta-analysis of motivational interviewing: Twenty-five years of empirical studies. *Research on Social Work Practice*, 20(2):137–160.

Magill M, Ray L (2009). Cognitive behavioural treatment with adult alcohol and illicit drug users: a meta-analysis of randomized controlled trials. *Journal of Studies on Alcohol and Drugs*, 70:516–527.

McCambridge J, Day M (2007). Randomized controlled trial of the effects of completing the Alcohol Use Disorders Identification Test questionnaire on self-reported hazardous drinking. *Addiction*, 103(2):241–248.

McCormick R et al. (2010). The research translation problem: alcohol screening and brief intervention in primary care – real world evidence supports theory. *Drugs: Education, Prevention and Policy*, 17(6):732–748s.

McQueen J et al. (2011). Brief interventions for heavy alcohol users admitted to general hospital wards. *Cochrane Database of Systematic Reviews*, (8):CD005191.

Miller W, Wilbourne P (2002). Mesa Grande: a methodological analysis of clinical trials of treatments for alcohol use disorders. *Addiction*, 97(3):265–277.

Moreira MT, Smith LA, Foxcroft D (2009). Social norms interventions to reduce alcohol misuse in university or college students (review). *Cochrane Database of Systematic Reviews*, (3):CD006748.

Moyer A, Finney JW, Swearingen CE (2002). Brief interventions for alcohol problems: a meta-analytic review of controlled investigations in treatment-seeking and non-treatment-seeking populations. *Addiction*, 97(3):279–292.

NICE (2010). *Alcohol-use disorders: preventing the development of hazardous and harmful drinking*. London, National Institute for Health and Clinical Excellence.

Nilsen P et al. (2008). A systematic review of emergency care brief alcohol interventions for injury patients. *Journal of Substance Abuse Treatment*, 35:184–201.

Peltzer K (2009). Brief intervention of alcohol problems in sub-Saharan Africa: a review. *Journal of Psychology in Africa*, 19(3):415–422.

Richmond R et al. (1995). Controlled evaluation of a general practice-based brief intervention for excessive drinking. *Addiction*, 90(1):119–132.

Richmond R et al. (2000). Evaluation of a workplace brief intervention for excessive alcohol consumption: the Workscreen project. *Preventive Medicine*, 30:51–63.

Riper H et al. (2009). Curbing problem drinking with personalised feedback interventions: a meta-analysis. *American Journal of Preventive Medicine*, 36:247–255.

Rooke S et al. (2010). Computer-delivered intervention for alcohol and tobacco use: a meta-analysis. *Addiction*, 105:1381–1390.

Rösner S et al. (2010a). Acamprosate for alcohol dependence. *Cochrane Database of Systematic Reviews*, (8):CD004332.

Rösner S et al. (2010b). Opioid antagonists for alcohol dependence. *Cochrane Database of Systematic Reviews*, (12):CD001867.

Saitz R (2010). Alcohol screening and brief intervention in primary care: absence of evidence for efficacy in people with dependence or very heavy drinking. *Drug and Alcohol Review*, 29:631–640.

Smedslund G et al. (2011). Motivational interviewing for substance abuse. *Cochrane Database of Systematic Reviews*, (5):CD008063.

Stade B et al. (2009). Psychological and/or educational interventions for reducing alcohol consumption in pregnant women and women planning pregnancy. *Cochrane Database of Systematic Reviews*, (2):CD004228.

Sullivan L et al. (2011). A meta-analysis of the efficacy of non-physician brief interventions for unhealthy alcohol use: implications for the patient-centered medical home. *American Journal on Addictions*, 20:343–356.

Tripodi S et al. (2010). Interventions for reducing adolescent alcohol abuse: a meta-analytic review. *Archives of Pediatric and Adolescent Medicine*, 164(1):85–91.

Vasilaki E, Hosier S, Cox W (2006). The efficacy of motivational interviewing as a brief intervention for excessive drinking: a meta-analytic review. *Alcohol and Alcoholism*, 41:328–335.

White A et al. (2010). Online alcohol interventions: a systematic review. *Journal of Medical Internet Research*, 12(5):e62.

Whitlock EP et al. (2004). Behavioral counseling interventions in primary care to reduce risky/harmful alcohol use by adults: a summary of the evidence for the US Preventive Services Task Force. *Annals of Internal Medicine*, 140:557–568.

WHO Regional Office for Europe (2009). *Evidence for the effectiveness and cost–effectiveness of interventions to reduce alcohol-related harm*. Copenhagen, WHO Regional Office for Europe (http://www.euro.who.int/__data/assets/pdf_file/0020/43319/E92823.pdf, accessed 12 February 2012).

Wilson G et al. (2011). Intervention against excessive alcohol consumption in primary health care: a survey of GPs' attitudes and practices in England ten years on. *Alcohol and Alcoholism*, 46(5):570–577.

Wutzke S et al. (2002). The long-term effectiveness of brief interventions for unsafe alcohol consumption: a 10-year follow-up. *Addiction*, 97:665–675.

Reducing injuries and death from alcohol-related road crashes

Francesco Mitis and Dinesh Sethi

Introduction

Road traffic injuries are a leading cause of death and a major public health problem in Europe as in the rest of the world. They decimate the lives of young people and result in enormous costs for families, emergency and health services and society at large (Peden et al., 2004; WHO Regional Office for Europe, 2009a). In the whole WHO European Region, road traffic injuries are the leading cause of death in children and young adults aged 5–29 years (WHO Regional Office for Europe, 2007). Alcohol use has been identified as one of the most important risk factors in the causation and severity of road traffic crashes. The consumption of alcohol, even in small doses, increases the risk of being involved in a road crash for all road users, whether motorists or pedestrians. This is because alcohol interferes with road users' skills by impairing cognition, vision and reaction time (Peden et al., 2004). It also increases the likelihood of adopting other risky forms of behaviour, such as speeding and not using safety equipment such as seat-belts and helmets.

At any blood alcohol concentration (BAC) greater than zero the risk of being involved in a crash rises. For the general driving population this risk rises significantly at levels higher than 0.4 g/litre (Peden et al., 2004). For motorcyclists with a BAC over 0.5 g/litre, the risk of having a crash is up to 40 times higher than with a zero BAC (WHO, 2007).

For inexperienced young adults and teenagers, the risks are even higher (Peden et al., 2004) and rise rapidly with an increasing BAC (WHO, 2007). At any BAC, drivers aged 16–20 years are three times more likely to crash than drivers who are older than 30 years (WHO, 2004). In the countries of the WHO European Region, road traffic injuries are the leading cause of death in children and young adults aged 5–29 years (Peden et al., 2004). However, although young people are at the greatest relative risk of having a drink–driving crash, in absolute terms drink–driving and related crashes and fatalities are more common among middle-aged people.

Summary of current evidence

There is wide evidence supporting the effectiveness of preventive interventions (Peden et al., 2004; WHO, 2007). Evidence indicates that for each euro invested in prevention carried out through random breath-testing, €36 could be saved (Racioppi et al., 2005).

The main conclusions from a recent comprehensive review (WHO Regional Office for Europe, 2009b) confirm and complement earlier findings.

There is consistent evidence that:

- the introduction (Mann et al., 2001) and/or reduction (Bernhoft & Behrensdorff, 2003; Bartl & Esberger, 2000; Shults et al., 2001) of legal BAC levels for driving, when these are enforced, reduce motor vehicle crashes and fatalities (Albalate, 2006);
- the introduction of sobriety checkpoints and random breath-testing reduces motor vehicle crashes and fatalities (Shults et al., 2001).

There is some evidence that motor vehicle crashes and fatalities can be reduced by:

- lower legal BAC levels for novice drivers (Shults et al., 2001; Hartling et al., 2004);
- licence suspension (Zobeck & Williams, 1994);
- brief advice and mandatory treatment of drivers with alcohol dependency;
- alcohol locks (Willis, Lybrand & Bellamy, 2004; Bjerre, 2005; Bjerre & Kostela, 2008; Bjerre & Thorsson, 2008);

and that mass media campaigns can be used to enhance the effectiveness of drink–driving policies (Elder et al., 2004).

There is no evidence that designated driver and safe ride programmes reduce motor vehicle crashes and fatalities (Ditter et al., 2005).

It is not known which are the most effective ways to ensure the existence of adequate and sustained resources to enforce legal BAC levels (WHO Regional Office for Europe, 2009b).

Deaths and injuries from road traffic crashes with alcohol a risk factor

Every year, approximately 43 500 people die on the roads in the EU (WHO Regional Office for Europe, 2009a) and many more are injured, with younger males more at risk. Vulnerable road users such as pedestrians, cyclists and users of motorized two-wheelers constitute 41% of all deaths. The burden is unevenly distributed: with few exceptions, it is more concentrated in the Baltic countries and in the central and eastern parts of the EU (Fig. 15) (WHO Regional Office for Europe, 2012b). Differences are, however, observed within countries too, with the poorest part of the population more at risk (WHO Regional Office for Europe, 2009a). The cost to countries has been estimated to be 2–3% of their GDP (WHO Regional Office for Europe, 2009a).

Attributable fractions of the mortality from road traffic injuries due to alcohol have been derived from several studies and summarized in a 2004 WHO publication which estimated the burden of disease attributable to selected major risk factors (Rehm et al., 2004). Based on a review of the literature globally, it is estimated that 33% of motor vehicle traffic injuries to males and 11% to females are due to alcohol (Ridolfo & Stevenson, 2001). For pedestrians, 40% of male and 17% of female deaths resulting from road traffic injuries are estimated to be due to alcohol (Ridolfo & Stevenson, 2001) while, for cyclists, the figures range from 20% for males (Single et al. 1999; Stinson et al., 1993) to 18% for females (English et al., 1995). The risk of road traffic deaths attributable to alcohol varies with age; in western European countries it has been estimated as 50% for males aged 30–44 years and 46% for those aged 15–29 years, and for females, 25% and 18%, respectively. In the Baltic and the central European countries these proportions are considerably higher (Rehm et al., 2004).

Estimates vary widely from country to country on the percentage of road traffic deaths attributable to alcohol. According to the data available, nine countries in the EU report that 20% or more (up to 48%) of road traffic deaths are attributable to alcohol, and a further six countries indicate that alcohol consumption causes 10–20% of fatalities. The information available is, however, incomplete, with only 85% of countries providing data (WHO Regional Office for Europe, 2009a), and its reliability will be influenced by the completeness and practice of BAC-testing in the event of a road crash. Information on crashes associated with raised BAC (Fig.16)

Fig. 15. Standardized mortality rates per 100 000 population from road traffic injuries in EU countries, Norway and Switzerland, 2010 (or most recently available)

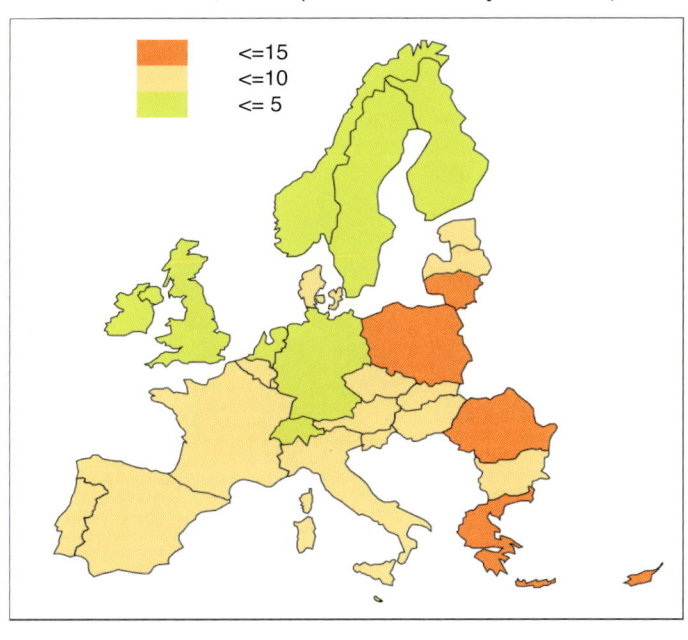

Source: European Health for All database, January 2012 (WHO Regional Office for Europe, 2012b).

is available in 93% of the countries belonging to the EU (WHO Regional Office for Europe, 2012b). These data need to be interpreted with caution because the completeness and frequency of testing for BAC levels in the event of a crash, enforcement levels of drink–driving laws and permissible BAC vary across countries. They are likely to underestimate the true prevalence of alcohol-related crashes.

The EU has supported a range of projects focused on alcohol and road safety (see Annex 4).

Conclusions for policy and practice

All EU countries have legislation that prohibits driving under the influence of alcohol. Four countries have set a limit of zero (WHO Regional Office for Europe, 2012a), but two countries have a legal BAC limit of 0.8 g/litre, above the level recommended by WHO and the EC of 0.5 g/litre. Despite the susceptibility of young drivers to crashing under the influence of alcohol, only half of the countries (14 out of 27) in the EU have set a BAC limit for young and novice drivers of 0.2 g/litre or below (WHO Regional Office for Europe, 2009a).

The range of countermeasures to reduce drink–driving implemented in EU countries was surveyed for a report on the implementation of the European Council recommendation on the prevention of injury and the promotion of safety and the Regional Committee resolution on prevention of injuries in the WHO European Region (WHO Regional Office for Europe, 2010a).

In 88% of the 25 EU countries that responded to the questionnaire, alcohol was identified as a risk factor for unintentional injuries in national policies. The vast majority had a national policy for road safety (96%) and were implementing (nationally or locally) interventions to prevent road traffic injuries (81%). For example, 87% had sobriety checkpoints but only seven countries

Fig.16. Road traffic crashes involving alcohol per 100 000 population in EU countries, Norway and Switzerland, quintiles, 2010

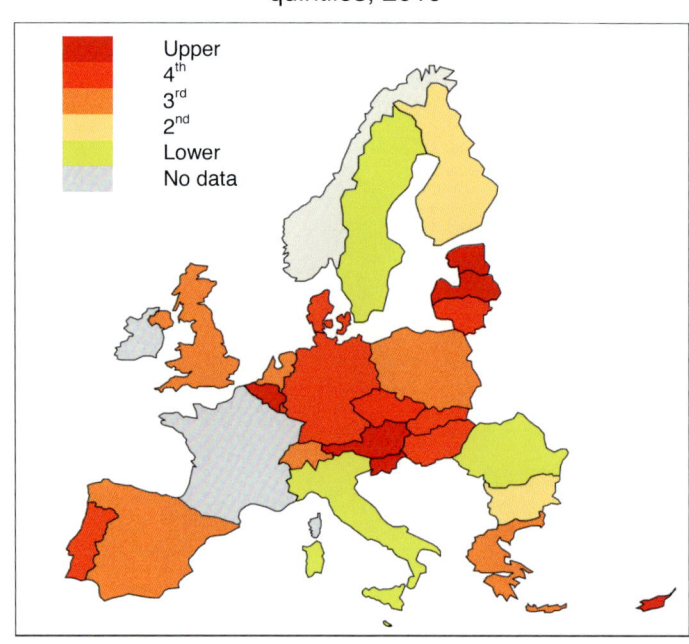

Source: European Health for All database, January 2012 (WHO Regional Office for Europe, 2012b).

applied restrictions on the sale of alcoholic beverages at petrol stations (WHO Regional Office for Europe, 2010b).

Although all countries have national policies on drink–driving, the lack of enforcement remains a critical issue. Of 23 EU country respondents, 16 (70%) indicated that the enforcement of drink–driving legislation was suboptimal. The importance of enforcement, notably through random breath-testing, has been highlighted by the EC (European Commission, 2004) and WHO alike (WHO Regional Office for Europe, 2010b; 2011b). Other countries have also reported that the penalties for drink–driving are insufficiently severe to act as a deterrent (WHO Regional Office for Europe, 2009a).

In order to reduce the mortality, morbidity and economic loss due to drink–driving, the following main points for action are proposed (WHO Regional Office for Europe, 2010b; 2011b):

- for any country with a BAC limit above 0.5 g/litre, it would be beneficial to reduce the level to 0.5 g/litre;
- in those countries with a BAC limit of 0.5 g/litre, additional benefit could be gained by reducing it to 0.2 g/litre;
- the legal BAC level for novice and professional drivers should be reduced to 0.2 g/litre or less;
- coverage of testing for BAC levels should be improved; and
- enforcement can be enhanced by increasing the use of random breath-testing and by increasing the fear of being caught; evidence shows that drivers need to know that there is a real risk of being stopped and breath-tested at any time.

As with many of the other alcohol policy issues discussed in this report, the key issue comes down to ensuring adequate implementation of what is known. Some countries have up-to-date alcohol-in-traffic laws and enforcement systems, and among countries with adequate measurement of BAC involvement, these countries do much better in holding down the number of crashes where alcohol is involved.

References

Albalate D (2006). *Lowering blood alcohol content levels to save lives: the European experience.* Barcelona, Research Institute of Applied Economics (No. CREAP20006-07).

Bartl G, Esberger R (2000). Effects of lowering the legal BAC-limit in Austria. *International Conference on Alcohol, Drugs and Traffic Safety, Stockholm, 22–26 May 2000.*

Bernhoft IM, Behrensdorff I (2003). Effect of lowering the alcohol limit in Denmark. *Accident Analysis and Prevention*, 35(4):515–525.

Bjerre B (2005). Primary and secondary prevention of drink–driving by the use of alcolock device and program: Swedish experiences. *Accident Analysis & Prevention*, 37(6):1145–1152.

Bjerre B, Kostela J (2008). Primary prevention of drink–driving by the large scale use of alcolocks in commercial vehicles. *Accident Analysis & Prevention*, 40(4):1294–1299.

Bjerre B, Thorsson U (2008). Is an alcohol ignition interlock programme a useful tool for changing the alcohol and driving habits of drink-drivers? *Accident Analysis & Prevention*, 40(1):267–273.

Ditter SM et al. (2005). Effectiveness of designated driver programs for reducing alcohol-impaired driving a systematic review. *American Journal of Preventive Medicine*, 28(Suppl. 5):280–287.

Elder RW et al. (2004). Effectiveness of mass media campaigns for reducing drinking and driving and alcohol-involved crashes: a systematic review. *American Journal of Preventive Medicine*, 27:57–65.

English D (1995). *The quantification of drug caused morbidity and mortality in Australia 1995.* Canberra, Commonwealth Department of Human Services and Health.

European Commission (2004). Commission recommendation of 6 April 2004 on enforcement in the field of road safety, 2004/345/EC. *Official Journal*, L 111/75.

Hartling L et al. (2004). Graduated driver licensing for reducing motor vehicle crashes among young drivers. *Cochrane Database of Systematic Reviews*, (2):CD003300.

Mann RE et al. (2001). The effects of introducing or lowering legal per se blood limits for driving: an international review. *Accident Analysis & Prevention*, 33:569–583.

Peden M et al., eds. (2004). *World report on road traffic injury prevention.* Geneva, World Health Organization.

Racioppi F et al., eds. (2005). *Preventing road traffic injury: a public health perspective for Europe.* Copenhagen, WHO Regional Office for Europe.

Rehm J et al. (2004). Alcohol use. In: Ezzati M, Lopez AD, Rodgers A, Murray CJL et al., eds. *Comparative quantification of health risks.* Geneva, World Health Organization:959–1108.

Ridolfo B, Stevenson C (2001). *The quantification of drug-caused mortality and morbidity in Australia 1998.* Canberra, Australian Institute of Health and Welfare.

Shults RA et al. (2001). Reviews of evidence regarding interventions to reduce alcohol-impaired driving. *American Journal of Preventive Medicine*, 21:66–88.

Single E et al. (1999). Morbidity and mortality attributable to alcohol, tobacco, and illicit drug use in Canada. *American Journal of Public Health*, 89:385–390.

Stinson FS et al. (1993). Alcohol-related mortality in the United States, 1979–1989. *Alcohol Health and Research World*, 17:251–260.

WHO (2007). *Drinking and driving. A road safety manual for decision-makers and practitioners.* Geneva, World Health Organization, Global Road Safety Partnership.

WHO Regional Office for Europe (2007). *Youth and road safety. Policy briefing* [web site]. Copenhagen, WHO Regional Office for Europe (http://www.euro.who.int/en/what-we-do/health-topics/disease-prevention/violence-and-injuries/publications/pre-2009/youth-and-road-safety-in-europe2.-policy-briefing, accessed 12 February 2012).

WHO Regional Office for Europe (2009a). *European status report on road safety* [web site]. Copenhagen, WHO Regional Office for Europe (http://www.euro.who.int/en/what-we-publish/abstracts/european-status-report-on-road-safety.-towards-safer-roads-and-healthier-transport-choices, accessed 12 February 2012).

WHO Regional Office for Europe (2009b). *Evidence for the effectiveness and cost–effectiveness of interventions to reduce alcohol-related harm.* Copenhagen, WHO Regional Office for Europe (http://www.euro.who.int/__data/assets/pdf_file/0020/43319/E92823.pdf, accessed 12 February 2012).

WHO Regional Office for Europe (2010a). Preventing injuries in Europe: from international collaboration to local implementation [web site]. Copenhagen, WHO Regional Office for Europe (http://www.euro.who.int/en/what-we-do/health-topics/disease-prevention/violence-and-injuries/publications/2010/preventing-injuries-in-europe-from-international-collaboration-to-local-implementation, accessed 12 February 2012).

WHO Regional Office for Europe (2010b). *European status report on alcohol and health 2010.* Copenhagen, WHO Regional Office for Europe (http://www.euro.who.int/en/what-we-do/health-topics/disease-prevention/alcohol-use/publications/2010/european-status-report-on-alcohol-and-health-2010, accessed 12 February 2012).

WHO Regional Office for Europe (2012a). Alcohol control database [online database]. Copenhagen, WHO Regional Office for Europe (http://data.euro.who.int/alcohol/Default.aspx?TabID=2422, accessed 12 February 2012).

WHO Regional Office for Europe (2012b). European Health for All database (HFA-DB) [online database]. Copenhagen, WHO Regional Office for Europe (http://www.euro.who.int/en/what-we-do/data-and-evidence/databases/european-health-for-all-database-hfa-db2, accessed 22 February 2012).

Willis C, Lybrand S, Bellamy N (2004). Alcohol ignition interlock programmes for reducing drink–driving recidivism. *Cochrane Database of Systematic Reviews*, (4):CD004168.

Zobeck TS, Williams GD (1994). *Evaluation synthesis of the impacts of DWI laws and enforcement methods: final report.* Rockville, MD, National Institute on Alcohol Abuse and Alcoholism, Office of Policy Analysis.

Community action

Allaman Allamani

Preventive intervention at the community level

The social, health and economic burdens from alcohol (as well as from tobacco and other drugs) have impacts at both national and local level, and effective interventions are, therefore, needed at each level. A community-based approach can contribute decisively to the success of different types of preventive intervention, increasing their probability of success through the resonance and enhancement provided by the local context.

Rather than focusing on vulnerable individuals or providing treatment for those afflicted, this approach involves a shift from the individual to the societal level. A central aspect of community work is the bottom-up approach and the sharing process, by which local people are considered active contributors to identifying problems and bringing about changes. The prevention expert's task would, therefore, be to give information about non-obvious problems which may be nested in the population, and to favour the expression of local needs, taking into account the readiness of the community to accept or to reframe the preventive initiatives. When the community is ready, the professional can mobilize local resources to increase health awareness and start preventive action. In doing so, he or she needs to connect with local stakeholders and the key people who coordinate local action and contribute to the coalition with the community's organizations and institutions.

In general, community interventions for alcohol-related problems consist of information/ education, enforcement of restrictive rules in existing legislation and mobilization of residents to create preventive initiatives. The *area* of the intervention can be, for example, a group of community schools, the retail sector and restaurants, the traffic sector and the local police, a holiday resort or the overall community.

The *evaluation* can address changes in knowledge (which are difficult to assess clearly in terms of effect on subsequent behaviour of the individuals informed), attitudes about risky behaviour and consumption, and rates of accidents, violence or deaths. Community-based prevention is difficult to evaluate, even when local government funding and involvement is available. Qualitative evaluation is necessary but will not suffice; testable hypotheses, a well-defined time frame, access to high-quality data and an evaluation design, preferably including control communities, are also required (Anderson & Baumberg, 2006).

One of the problems with the scientific literature on community action is that it tends to be positive-thinking and convinced that whatever is done is worthwhile. However, the basic conclusion drawn from community action that has shown an effect is that it was directed at concrete goals, mainly reducing drink–driving casualties, assaults or underage drinking. The involvement of community actors provides a cover and level of acceptance in the community, but what actually works is regulatory enforcement of one kind or another, mainly directed at those who serve alcohol, although sometimes also at drinkers (for example, enforcement of drink–driving regulations).

Successful alcohol preventive community programmes have been implemented in Canada and the United States since the 1970s (Giesbrecht et al., 1990; Greenfield & Zimmerman, 1993), and a decade later they were also implemented in a few European countries (Holmila, 1997; Larsson & Hanson, 1997; WHO Regional Office for Europe, 1999). Their relative diffusion in Europe was supported by the publication of the WHO European Alcohol Action Plan in 1992 (WHO Regional Office for Europe, 1992), which recommended local action as an important prevention approach. The Malmö community-based study, undertaken during the 1970s in Sweden, was the first European community action project, and it was able to demonstrate that under the right conditions, the positive effects on health can be dramatic. An intervention for heavy drinkers consisting of early identification and brief information, backed up with periodic control of blood gamma-GT, resulted in half the number of deaths that occurred in the control group which did not receive the intervention at six-year follow-up (Kristenson et al., 1983).

Almost all the European countries recently reported that community prevention is part of their current alcohol policy (WHO, 2010; WHO Regional Office for Europe, 2010). This may be an overestimation since, according to data from the ongoing EU-funded Alcohol Measures for Public Health Research Alliance (AMPHORA) project in 2010, only 7 out of 12 countries have community projects aimed at reducing alcohol-related problems (AMPHORA, 2011).

The two most recent and significant books which summarize the available evidence for the new alcohol policies are the *Evidence for the effectiveness and cost–effectiveness of interventions to reduce alcohol-related harm* (WHO Regional Office for Europe, 2009) and the second edition of *Alcohol: no ordinary commodity* (Babor et al., 2010). Both publications concluded that projects based on information do not produce visible changes, even if they can increase knowledge. On the other hand, those that actively involve and mobilize the local population and its organizational forms in different sectors (including the enforcement of existing norms such as prohibition of sales to minors, responsible beverage service and control of drink–driving) can not only increase citizens' knowledge about and attitudes towards the risks of their own drinking, but also limit their purchase and consumption of alcohol and drinking before driving, and eventually reduce alcohol-related harm such as violence and traffic fatalities.

Some recent initiatives have the merit of introducing the community action approach in areas where little prevention work was previously done. Examples are a multi-year community action project in South Tyrol, Italy, about preventive measures to enhance awareness in dealing with alcohol and drugs among children and adolescents as well as their parents (Greca, Schäfferling &, Siebenhüter, 2009); some community programmes in Denmark oriented towards minimizing harm and focusing on risky situations and areas (Elmeland, 2006); and attempts to replicate the United States study of three community trials (Holder et al., 2000) in three United Kingdom cities in 2003 (Hodgson & Davidson, 2008), adopting a community partnership approach.

Programmes that spread public health information about the risk of alcohol can also focus individuals' attention on their own drinking behaviour. An "Alcohol, less is better" community-based prevention programme was carried out in Italy from 1999 to 2006, designed as a controlled intervention trial (Bagnardi et al., 2011). The intervention had the collaboration of community leaders and institutional or volunteer organizations in 10 selected small Italian communities involving more than 100 000 individuals, with the aim of informing and sensitizing the community about the harmful effects of alcohol. Eight communities were chosen as a control group. Overall, a significant reduction in individual self-reported alcohol consumption before and after the intervention was observed in the intervention sample (-1.1 drinks/week) relative to the control sample (+0.3 drinks/week).

Generally, projects that are able to *mobilize the community* and activate its various components, including community members and organizations, and promote grassroots initiatives have been shown to produce different types of positive change in the local population, such as changed attitudes towards alcohol sales to minors, wider acceptance of public health material, the sharing of local initiatives to promote healthy lifestyles, reduced alcohol consumption and reduced drunkenness. The following are some examples.

- A programme in a holiday resort in the Netherlands during 2004, which involved representatives of the municipality and of the stakeholders who have a role in dealing with excessive alcohol use, was able to increase the attention given to sales to minors and to reduce the nuisance to third parties (van de Luitgaarden, Knibbe & Wiers, 2010).

- A multicomponent community project in Scandicci, Italy, which in 2000–2003 involved several hundred residents (schoolchildren and members of community organizations) in producing and distributing information material locally, gradually increased the awareness of the risks of alcohol in a culture that traditionally has a strong positive attitude towards drinking (Allamani et al., 2007).

- A campaign to distribute health information pamphlets during the delivery of a brief intervention programme to health professionals in Tampere, Finland, which was supported by a community-based approach, turned out to be successful at least in terms of visibility of the material delivered (Kääriäinen et al., 2008).

- A project in Sweden aimed at supporting the local community through a local coordinating committee, which formulated and implemented interventions to reduce heavy episodic drinking and to delay the onset age of alcohol consumption (the 1996–2002 Trelleborg project), was able to show a considerable decrease in alcohol consumption among those adolescents who were excessive drinkers (Stafström et al., 2006; Stafström & Östergren, 2008).

- A quasi-experimental two-and-a-half-year alcohol prevention programme addressed at 900 schoolchildren aged 13–16 years in Örebro, Sweden, and also aiming to influence parents' attitudes towards underage drinking, demonstrated at post-test that young people in the intervention group reported less drunkenness and delinquency (Koutakis, Stattin & Kerr, 2008).

Other multicomponent projects, which included such initiatives as responsible beverage service and stricter enforcement of drink–driving regulations and sales norms, were able to demonstrate reductions in sales to minors and intoxicated patrons as well as in the illegal availability of alcohol, alcohol-related violence, car crashes and even deaths. Examples are given below.

- A multicomponent community intervention to reduce the number of sales to intoxicated individuals and subsequent alcohol-related violence and injuries (Local Alcohol Policy project, or PAKKA in Finnish) was conducted in the Finnish town of Jyväskylä between 2004 and 2007 (Warpenius & Holmila, 2010). A local multi-agency steering group and a working group developed the intervention with the following components: enforcement of norms about liquor licensing, a training programme for alcohol servers, community mobilization and campaigns to reinforce policies and media coverage. In the evaluation, refusal of service to a pseudo-drunk customer significantly increased in the intervention area from 23% in 2004 to 42% in 2007.

- A 10-year Swedish multicomponent programme was also conducted in Stockholm starting in 1996 and based on community mobilization, training in responsible beverage service for servers and stricter enforcement of existing alcohol laws. Data on police-reported violence during the period January 1994 to September 2000 showed a 29% reduction in violent crimes in the intervention area compared with the control area (Wallin, Norstrom & Andreasson, 2001).

- The goal of the quasi-experimental Sacramento Neighbourhood Alcohol Prevention Project in California was the reduction of access to alcohol, drinking and related problems in two low-income predominantly ethnic minority neighbourhoods. The focus was on individuals aged 15–29 years (Treno et al., 2007), with the Sacramento community at large as the control site. The five components of the intervention carried out between 2001 and 2003 included mobilization, community awareness, responsible beverage service, and enforcement of the law on access to alcohol by minors and the law on intoxicated patrons. The results demonstrated the effectiveness of interventions in terms of sales of alcohol to minors, and a reduction in alcohol-related problems such as assaults and motor vehicle crashes.

Community action programmes are implemented within the overall context of national developments and policies which may delimit the scope of action or moderate the effects.

One such was a large community trial conducted in six urban and rural municipalities (and six control communities) in Sweden during 2003–2006, where activities took place with alcohol and drug coordinators at the county level and local coordinators at the municipal level (Kvillemo, Andréasson & Bränström, 2008). The focus of the action plan was to stimulate evidence-based preventive measures at the municipal level in order to reduce problems related to alcohol and drug use. The positive outcomes of the project were: increased commitment and cooperation by local politicians, administrators, police and general practitioners; more responsible beverage service, with less alcohol served to minors in bars and restaurants (a decrease from about 45% in 1997 to about 15% in 2007); and a reduction in the social and illegal availability of alcohol. The communities gradually reoriented their thinking about prevention from a single focus on youth activities to a broader approach involving the whole population. However, after an initial surge, alcohol consumption levels stabilized after 2004, and other problem indicators such as hospital admissions for alcohol intoxication among teenagers, as well as crime indicators, indicate that the alcohol situation developed negatively during the implementation period. These trends might be explained by other non-prevention factors occurring in the meantime, such as a decrease in the price of alcohol, an increase in import allowances and more premises licensed to sell alcohol beverages.

Only a few studies have estimated the *costs* of community action projects or the cost savings achieved. If only mass media campaigns are considered, these interventions are not expensive (Chisholm, 2004). In the Stockholm project on training in responsible beverage service implemented since 1996 (Wallin, Norstrom & Andreasson, 2001), a cost–saving ratio of 1:39 was reached, considering the costs of both the programme (about €796 000) and of violent crimes (Mansdotter et al., 2007).

A systematic review was conducted to determine the effectiveness and economic efficiency of multicomponent programmes with community mobilization for reducing alcohol-impaired driving (Shults et al., 2009). Six studies published between 1994 and 2002 (Rhode Island Department of Health, 1994; Hingson et al., 1996; 2005; Holder et al., 2000; Wagenaar, Murray & Toomey, 2000; Voas et al., 2002) qualified for the review. According to evidence, carefully planned multicomponent programmes (including efforts to limit access to alcohol, particularly among young people, training in responsible beverage service, sobriety checkpoints, public education and media advocacy), when implemented in conjunction with community mobilization efforts, are effective in reducing alcohol-related road crashes.

Three studies have reported evidence that such programmes produce cost savings. A study in Massachusetts, United States (Hingson et al., 1996) showed that the 26 alcohol-related deaths averted as a result of the programme resulted in savings of approximately US$ 20 million – an estimated saving of US$ 9.33 for each dollar invested. The Community Trials Project (Holder et al., 2000) returned an estimated US$ 6.56 in savings for every dollar invested, while the Community Trials Project comparative study in Salinas, California returned an estimated US$ 15.72 in savings for each dollar invested.

Table 7 summarizes the evidence of the impact of community projects on alcohol published since 2006.

Table 7. Summary of evidence on alcohol community projects published since 2006

Area of project	Evidence
Information/ education and the community	Of the 20 trials included in a Cochrane review of studies on the effectiveness of multicomponent prevention programmes with a combination of school, community and/or family-based interventions in preventing alcohol misuse in school-aged children up to 18 years of age (Foxcroft & Tsertsvadze, 2011), 12 showed some evidence of effectiveness in terms of reductions in alcohol use or heavy drinking compared to a control or other intervention group, with effects lasting from 3 months to 3 years.
Drink–driving and the community	A systematic review was conducted to determine the effectiveness and economic efficiency of multicomponent programmes with community mobilization for reducing alcohol-impaired driving (Shults et al., 2009).According to evidence in the six studies which qualified for review, carefully planned, multicomponent programmes (including efforts to limit access to alcohol, particularly among young people, training in responsible service of beverages, sobriety checkpoints, public education and media advocacy), when implemented in conjunction with community mobilization efforts, are effective in reducing alcohol-related road crashes. Three studies reported evidence that such programmes produce cost savings.
Mobilization and multiple interventions within the community	Projects that are able to mobilize the community and activate its components, as well as community members and organizations, have been shown to produce different types of positive change in the local population, including changed attitudes towards alcohol sales to minors, sharing local initiatives to promote healthy lifestyles, reduced alcohol consumption and reduced drunkenness. When these projects also focused on responsible beverage service and included stricter enforcement of drink–driving and sale norms, they were able to demonstrate reductions of sales to minors or to intoxicated patrons, reductions in illegal availability of alcohol (as in the case of the Swedish six community trial), and a decrease in alcohol-related violence and car crashes (as in the Sacramento study).

Conclusions

Community action to prevent alcohol-related harm is an important area where science can interact with citizens and allow for shared and practical initiatives to improve the public health. Community projects work best when they mobilize different sectors of the community. A community approach can also be a successful support for different alcohol preventive programmes.

To prevent the reduction or disappearance of successful outcomes over time after the end of the project, alcohol (and other drug) community action programmes should also include the means to institutionalize effective prevention efforts, which can be done in cooperation with the local authorities (Holder, 2010).

A consistent and coordinated relationship between local and national initiatives should be sought, and caution should be exercised in transferring specific community programmes developed in one culture or setting to another. They may work well in one context and culture and less well in others where, in any case, they may have a degree of success from different perspectives, such as raising awareness to bring about popular acceptance of certain policies or changes in consumption (Andréasson, 2010).

Community action and prevention programmes have been criticized as being hardly a science (Gorman, 2010). To meet this criticism, efforts should be made to have programme evaluated by independent scholars so as to ascertain the extent to which the results reported are dependent on the analysis strategies employed by the original investigators.

References

Allamani A et al. (2007). Preliminary evaluation of the educational strategy of a community alcohol use action research project in Scandicci, Italy. *Substance Use & Misuse,* 42:2029–2040.

AMPHORA. The AMPHORA project [web site] (2010). Brussels, European Commission (http://amphora project.net, accessed 13 February 2012).

Anderson P, Baumberg B (2006). *Alcohol in Europe: a public health perspective.* London, Institute of Alcohol Studies.

Andréasson S (2010). Premature adoption and dissemination of prevention programmes. *Addiction,* 105(4): 583–584.

Babor TF et al. (2010). *Alcohol: no ordinary commodity. Research and public policy,* 2nd ed. Oxford, Oxford University Press.

Bagnardi V et al. (2011). 'Alcohol, less is better' project: outcomes of an Italian community-based prevention programme on reducing per-capita alcohol consumption. *Addiction,* 106(1):102–110.

Chisholm D et al. (2004). Reducing the global burden of hazardous alcohol use: a comparative cost–effectiveness analysis. *Journal of Studies on Alcohol and Drugs,* 65(6): 782–793.

Elmeland, K (2006). To prevent alcohol- and drug-related problems by community actions in Denmark. In: *Drug prevention, treatment and the media. Nordic perspective. Collection of essays on selected issues.* Tallin, Estonian Foundation for Prevention of Drug Addiction.

Foxcroft DR, Tsertsvadze A (2011). Universal multi-component prevention programs for alcohol misuse in young people. *Cochrane Database of Systematic Reviews,* (9):CD009307.

Giesbrecht N et al., eds. (1990). *Research, action and the community: experiences in the prevention of alcohol and other drug problems.* Rockville, MD, Office for Substance Abuse Prevention (OSAP Prevention Monograph 4) (http://www.eric.ed.gov/ERICWebPortal/search/detailmini.jsp?_nfpb=true&_& ERICExtSearch_SearchValue_0=ED333281&ERICExtSearch_SearchType_0=no&accno=ED333281, accessed 13 February 2012).

Gorman DM (2010). Understanding prevention research as a form of pseudoscience. *Addiction,* 105(4): 582–583.

Greca R, Schäfferling S, Siebenhüter S (2009). *Gefährdung Jugendlicher durch Alkohol und Drogen: Eine Fallstudie zur Wirksamkeit von Präventionsmaßnahmen [Vulnerability of young people to alcohol and drugs: a case study on the effectiveness of prevention measures].* Wiesbaden, VS Verlag für Sozialwissenschaften.

Greenfield TK, Zimmerman R, eds. (1993). *Experiences with community action projects: new research in the prevention of alcohol and other* problems. Rockville, MD, Center for Substance Abuse Prevention, Department of Health and Human Services (CSAP Prevention Monograph 14).

Hingson R et al. (1996). Reducing alcohol-impaired driving in Massachusetts: the Saving Lives Program. *American Journal of Public Health*, 86(6):791–797.

Hingson RW et al. (2005). Effects on alcohol related fatal crashes of a community based initiative to increase substance abuse treatment and reduce alcohol availability. *Injury Prevention*, 11(2):84–90.

Hodgson R, Davidson R (2008). UKCAPP: An Alcohol Education & Research Council initiative. *Drugs: Education, Prevention and Policy*, 15(S1):1–3.

Holder HH et al. (2000). Effect of community-based interventions on high-risk drinking and alcohol-related injuries. *Journal of the American Medical Association*, 284:2341–2347.

Holder HH (2010). Prevention programs in the 21st century: what we do not discuss in public. *Addiction*, 105(4):578–581.

Holmila M, ed. (1997). *Community prevention of alcohol problems*. London, Palgrave Macmillan.

Kääriäinen J, Aalto M, Kääriäinen M (2008). Audit questionnaire as part of community action against heavy drinking. *Alcohol and Alcoholism*, 43(4):442–445.

Koutakis N, Stattin H, Kerr M (2008). Reducing youth alcohol drinking through a parent-targeted intervention: the Örebro Prevention Program. *Addiction*, 103(10):1629–1637.

Kristenson H et al. (1983). Identification and intervention of heavy drinking in middle-aged men. Results and follow-up of 24–60 months of longterm study with randomised controls. *Alcoholism: Clinical and Experimental Research,* 7:203–209.

Kvillemo P, Andreasson S, Bränström R (2008). *Effekter av lokalt alkohol- och narkotikaförebyggande Arbete Utvärdering av det förebyggande arbetet i sex försökskommuner Huvudrapport [Effects of local alcohol and drug prevention work. Evaluation of the preventive work in six experimental municipalities. Main report]*. Östersund, Swedish National Institute of Public Health.

Larsson S, Hanson B, eds. (1997). *Community based alcohol prevention in Europe – methods and strategies*. Lund, Lund University, Studentlitteratur.

Mansdotter AM et al. (2007). A cost–effectiveness analysis of alcohol prevention targeting licensed premises. *European Journal of Public Health*, 17:618–623.

Rhode Island Department of Health (1994). *Final report of the Rhode Island Community Alcohol Abuse and Injury Prevention Project. Vol. I, technical report*. Providence, RI, Rhode Island Department of Health.

Shults RA et al. (2009). Effectiveness of multicomponent programs with community mobilization for reducing alcohol-impaired driving. *American Journal of Preventive Medicine*, 37(4):360–371.

Stafström M, Östergren PO (2008). A community-based intervention to reduce alcohol-related accidents and violence in 9th grade students in southern Sweden: the example of the Trelleborg project. *Accident Analysis & Prevention*, 40(3):920–925.

Stafström M et al. (2006). A community action program for reducing harmful drinking behaviour among adolescents: the Trelleborg project. *Addiction*, 101:813–823.

Treno AJ et al. (2007). The Sacramento Neighborhood Alcohol Prevention Project: outcomes from a community prevention trial. *Journal of Studies on Alcohol and Drugs*, 68(2):197–207.

van de Luitgaarden J, Knibbe R, Wiers RW (2010). Adolescents binge drinking when on holiday: an evaluation of a community intervention based on self-regulation. *Substance Use & Misuse,* 45(1–2):190–203.

Voas RB et al. (2002). Operation Safe Crossing: using science within a community intervention. *Addiction*, 97:1205–1214.

Wagenaar AC, Murray DM, Toomey TL (2000). Communities mobilizing for change on alcohol (CMCA): effects of a randomized trial on arrests and traffic crashes. *Addiction*, 95(2):209–217.

Wallin E, Norstrom T, Andreasson S (2001). Alcohol prevention targeting licensed premises: a study of effects on violence. *Journal of Studies on Alcohol and Drugs*, 72:723–730.

Warpenius K, Holmila M, Mustonen H (2010). Effects of a community intervention to reduce the serving of alcohol to intoxicated patrons. *Addiction*, 105:1032–1040.

WHO (2010). *Atlas on substance use. Resources for the prevention and treatment of substance use disorders.* Geneva, World Health Organization.

WHO Regional Office for Europe (1992). *European Alcohol Action Plan 1992–1999.* Copenhagen, WHO Regional Office for Europe.

WHO Regional Office for Europe (1999). *Community action to prevent alcohol problems.* Copenhagen, WHO Regional Office for Europe (http://www.euro.who.int/__data/assets/pdf_file/0003/119181/E63694.pdf, accessed 13 February 2012).

WHO Regional Office for Europe (2009). *Evidence for the effectiveness and cost–effectiveness of interventions to reduce alcohol-related harm.* Copenhagen, WHO Regional Office for Europe (http://www.euro.who.int/__data/assets/pdf_file/0020/43319/E92823.pdf, accessed 12 February 2012).

WHO Regional Office for Europe (2010). *European status report on alcohol and health 2010.* Copenhagen, WHO Regional Office for Europe.

Drinking environments

Karen Hughes, Mark A Bellis

Introduction

Pubs, bars and nightclubs are key locations for the consumption of alcohol, particularly among young people. These drinking venues can form a major part of individuals' social and recreational life, providing opportunities for fun, socializing, relaxation and physical exercise. They can also provide benefits to local economies including through employment, economic investment, regeneration and tourism. However, the congregation of large numbers of drinkers in drinking environments (defined here as public drinking venues and the areas surrounding them) means they are often associated with high levels of intoxication and alcohol-related harm, including violence, road traffic crashes, public disorder and unintentional injury (Bellis et al., 2010; Wahl, Kriston & Berner, 2010; Rowe et al., 2010). Alcohol-related problems typically cluster in areas with high numbers of pubs, bars and nightclubs and peak at weekend nights, along with alcohol-related emergency department attendances and crime (Gmel et al., 2005; Ricci et al., 2008; Livingston, Chikritzhs & Room, 2007; Grubesic & Pridemore, 2011). Further, studies show that a small number of drinking venues within an area often account for a large proportion of alcohol-related harm, suggesting that certain features of these premises can aggravate problem behaviour (Rowe et al., 2010; Hughes et al., 2011b). Key features of problematic venues include a permissive atmosphere, crowding, low levels of comfort, poorly trained staff and cheap drinks promotions (Hughes et al., 2011b; Graham et al., 2006; Graham & Homel, 2008). In addition to factors associated with drinking venues, the wider drinking environment surrounding pubs, bars and nightclubs can influence levels of harm (for example, the availability of public transport), as can cultural and societal factors, including drinking patterns. For example, recent studies show that many young Europeans consume alcohol at home or in streets and other public places before visiting pubs, bars and nightclubs (known as preloading or predrinking), with a general trend towards increasing purchases of alcohol off-premise[4] being seen across Europe.

The propensity for alcohol-related harm in drinking environments makes these settings key areas for interventions, which can seek to affect the way in which alcohol is served and the conditions in which it is consumed. Successful interventions can help to prevent risky behaviour, protect the health of individuals who socialize and work in drinking environments, and prevent the broader impacts on communities (such as vandalism) and society (such as work absenteeism) that can follow a night out.

A trend being observed in many European alcohol markets is a shift from the purchase of alcohol in on-premises (pubs, bars and nightclubs) to off-premises (such as supermarkets and liquor stores). Research by RAND Europe (Rabinovich et al., 2011) found that in four out of six countries studied (Finland, Germany, Ireland, Latvia, Slovenia and Spain), the proportion of alcohol consumption accounted for by off-premise purchases increased between 1997 and 2010 relative to the proportion accounted for by on-premise purchases. Changes were particularly pronounced in Ireland, where off-premise alcohol consumption increased by 72% over this

---

[4] In this report, "on-premise" sales and/or drinking of alcohol refers to premises, licensed or not, where drinking is permitted in the same place as the sales are made. "Off-premise" refers to places where sales are permitted but drinking is not, such as supermarkets.

period and on-premise consumption decreased by 56% (a 32% decrease overall). The share of total alcohol consumption accounted for by off-premise purchases increased from just 18% in 1997 to 47% in 2010. Increasing ratios of off- to on-premises were also identified in Spain (where alcohol consumption in licensed premises is still dominant) and in Finland and Germany (where off-premise consumption has traditionally exceeded drinking in licensed establishments).

One of the main reasons for this shift from consumption from on- to off-premises is thought to be the cheaper price of alcohol in off-premises, particularly in supermarkets. Surveys suggest that alcohol prices in licensed premises are typically around three times higher than those in the off-premise trade (Rabinovich et al., 2009). A general movement towards off-premise consumption suggests that home drinking is increasing and that less alcohol is being consumed in pubs, bars and nightclubs. While this may suggest that fewer people are using drinking environments, a growing body of research among young people shows that many consume alcohol bought from off-premises prior to visiting pubs, bars and nightclubs (Bellis et al., 2010; Wahl, Kriston & Berner, 2010; Hughes et al., 2011a; Forsyth, 2010; Hughes et al., 2008). For example, a study of 16–30-year-olds in drinking environments in four European cities (in the Netherlands, Slovenia, Spain and the United Kingdom) found that between 35% (Slovenia) and 61% (United Kingdom) of respondents had preloaded on the night they were surveyed (Hughes et al., 2011a). In Spain, 26% of participants had consumed alcohol at home and a further 34% had participated in *botellón* (group drinking in streets and other public settings) prior to visiting bars and nightclubs. Preloading is likely to have important implications for the management of drinking environments. For example, individuals may already be intoxicated when they arrive in drinking environments, or unable to consume more than a few drinks before becoming intoxicated. Serving alcohol to intoxicated individuals is illegal in most European countries, although enforcement levels vary and prosecutions can be rare (Bellis & Hughes, 2011). Thus, preloading may lead to fewer legal sales in bars yet more intoxication and alcohol-related problems, with studies suggesting that it can be associated with higher overall alcohol consumption on a night out and greater involvement in violence (Wahl, Kriston & Berner, 2010; Hughes et al., 2008). Fewer alcohol sales may also lead to greater use of cheap alcohol promotions in licensed premises as bars compete for customers, and to reduced spending and vigilance elsewhere (on, for example, staff training and responsible beverage service). Thus, understanding trends in preloading will be an important consideration when intervening in drinking environments to prevent alcohol-related harm.

Summary of recent evidence

During the last two to three years, a series of reviews (Brennan et al., 2011; Jones et al., 2011; WHO Regional Office for Europe, 2009; Babor et al., 2010; Ker & Chinnock, 2008; Bolier et al., 2011) and new studies have examined evidence of the impacts of interventions in drinking environments. These are summarized in Table 8.

Studies of *responsible beverage service training* continue to show limited evidence of effectiveness. A systematic review (Ker & Chinnock, 2008) concluded that there was inconclusive evidence for the impacts of interventions in alcohol server settings on patrons' alcohol consumption, conflicting evidence for such impacts on servers' behaviour, and insufficient evidence to suggest that they reduced injury. Only one study in the review had been published since 2006 (Toomey et al., 2008). This found an initial decrease in sales to pseudo-intoxicated patrons following a training programme for owners/managers of licensed premises in the United States, although the effects had disappeared after three months. Similar results have since been found in a follow-up study of responsible beverage service training for staff in student

Table 8. Summary of evidence published since 2006

Activity	Evidence
Responsible beverage service training	While responsible beverage service training can change servers' knowledge, there is insufficient evidence to support its effectiveness in changing their behaviour or reducing alcohol use and harm. New studies have shown that any initial benefits of RBS training effects can rapidly disappear.
Enforcement of on-premise regulations	Enforcement is critical to the success of interventions in drinking environments. New studies from Finland and the United Kingdom provide further support for the effectiveness of targeted enforcement activity in reducing irresponsible alcohol service and violence.
Server liability	A systematic review found strong evidence that server liability laws reduce alcohol-related harm. However, such laws are rare outside North America.
Safer drinking environments	Evidence suggests that interventions may reduce harm in drinking environments but do not address excessive alcohol use. In Australia, the use of security measures in drinking settings had no impact on alcohol-related injury.

bars in Sweden, where initial reductions in patrons' breath alcohol concentration (Johnsson & Berglund, 2003) were not sustained at five-month follow up (Johnsson & Berglund, 2009). In Finland, a study evaluating the PAKKA (Local Alcohol Policy) community intervention (Warpenius, Holmila & Mustonen, 2010) found that a responsible beverage service component had no independent effects on servers' practice, despite the overall programme having positive impacts on their behaviour (see below). In the United States, a responsible beverage service programme focusing on discouraging alcohol service to pregnant customers was used among staff from drinking premises in two states. An evaluation found that the refusal of service to pseudo-pregnant actors significantly increased following the training in one state, but that the programme had no impact in the other state (Dresser et al., 2011).

A 2006 report stressed that ongoing enforcement was critical to the success of responsible beverage service and other interventions in drinking environments (Anderson & Baumberg, 2006). New evidence supports this claim. In the evaluation of the PAKKA project in Finland (Warpenius, Holmila & Mustonen, 2010), improvements seen in refusal of service to pseudo-intoxicated actors were considered a result of a combination of increased surveillance and sanctions. In the United Kingdom, a study evaluating the use of combined police and emergency department data to target enforcement activity in drinking environments, including multi-agency enforcement in problem venues, found the intervention to be associated with reductions in hospital admissions for violence (Florence et al., 2011). Increases in less serious assaults recorded by police were also seen, and these were thought to be due to increased opportunities for reporting and detecting crimes. The strong evidence identified in 2006 for the effectiveness of *server liability* laws in reducing alcohol-related harm has been clarified though a new systematic review (Rammohan et al., 2011), although evidence remains limited to North America.

Some new evidence has been published regarding the impacts of *safer bar environments*, which aim to reduce harm without affecting alcohol consumption (Anderson & Baumberg, 2006). For example, studies of the use of safer drinking containers (polycarbonate glassware) in bars have found this to be feasible and have the potential to reduce injury (Anderson et al., 2009; Forsyth, 2008). Appraisals of broader safety and security measures in drinking environments have, however, been less positive. A study in Australia (Miller et al., 2011) found that a multicomponent intervention focusing on safety in drinking environments had no impact on alcohol-related emergency department attendances for injury. The programme included high-visibility policing, a safer drinking campaign and the use of closed circuit security cameras, a radio communication system linking security staff and police, and ID scanners in bars. Analyses found injury attendances continued to increase during the programme. Associations were identified between the implementation of both ID scanners and the drinking campaign and increased injury attendances, although these were considered coincidental rather than causal. An appraisal of measures to improve safety in United Kingdom drinking environments stressed that these are resource-intensive and have little impact on intoxication (Bellis & Hughes, 2011). Both this and the Australian study suggested a broader focus was required that sought to affect alcohol consumption rather than just manage its harms.

Since 2006, the EU has supported a range of projects focusing on reducing harm in drinking environments (see Annex 4).

Conclusions for policy and practice

The evidence base assessing the effectiveness of interventions in drinking environments has grown since 2006. New studies of responsible beverage service training have continued to find it to have limited impact, with any initial benefits short-lived. The evidence supporting enforcement activity in drinking premises has, however, increased. Studies examining measures to create safer drinking environments show mixed results, with one study in Australia finding that the introduction of a variety of security-focused interventions had no benefits in reducing alcohol-related injuries. The types of intervention assessed in this study (for example, high-visibility policing, CCTV, radio communications systems, ID scanners) are rare in most European countries, and largely represent attempts to control violence and disorder in areas where intoxication and related harm in drinking environments is already a major problem. An appraisal of similar measures implemented in United Kingdom drinking environments suggested that without tackling the underlying causes of intoxication, such measures aim only to create drinking environments where it is "safe" for individuals to get drunk. Here, however, the concept of safety does not consider the risks associated with drunkenness once people have left managed drinking environments, and ignores long-term health damages relating to repeated drunkenness.

Much evidence on interventions to create safer drinking environments focuses on settings where drunkenness and antisocial behaviour are endemic. Consequently, research is urgently required to identify those aspects of policy and practice that prevent such cultures developing in the first place and to understand the transferability of interventions developed for intoxicated nightlife environments to settings still characterized by more moderate drinking behaviour. The current diversity in drinking and nightlife cultures in Europe presents a key opportunity for developing this evidence base.

References

Anderson P, Baumberg B (2006). *Alcohol in Europe: a public health perspective*. London, Institute of Alcohol Studies.

Anderson Z et al. (2009). *Evaluation of the Lancashire polycarbonate glass pilot project*. Liverpool, Centre for Public Health, Liverpool John Moores University.

Babor TF et al. (2010). *Alcohol: no ordinary commodity. Research and public policy,* 2nd ed. Oxford, Oxford University Press.

Bellis MA et al. (2010). Cross-sectional measures and modelled estimates of blood alcohol levels in United Kingdom nightlife and their relationships with drinking behaviours and observed signs of inebriation. *Substance Abuse Treatment, Prevention, and Policy*, 5:5.

Bellis MA, Hughes K (2011). Getting drunk safely? Night-life policy in the United Kingdom and its public health consequences. *Drug and Alcohol Review*, 30(5):536–545.

Bolier L et al. (2011). Alcohol and drug prevention in nightlife settings: a review of experimental studies. *Substance Use & Misuse*, 46:1569–1591.

Brennan I et al. (2011). Interventions for disorder and severe intoxication in and around licensed premises, 1989–2009. *Addiction*, 106(4):706–713.

Dresser J et al. (2011). Field trial of alcohol-server training for prevention of fetal alcohol syndrome. *Journal of Studies on Alcohol and Drugs*, 72(3):490–496.

Florence C et al. (2011). Effectiveness of anonymised information sharing and use in health service, police, and local government partnership for preventing violence related injury: experimental study and time series analysis. *British Medical Journal*, 342:d3313.

Forsyth AJM (2008). Banning glassware from nightclubs in Glasgow (Scotland): observed impacts, compliance and patron's views. *Alcohol and Alcoholism*, 43(1):111–117.

Forsyth AJM (2010). Front, side, and back-loading: patrons' rationales for consuming alcohol purchased off-premises before, during, or after attending nightclubs. *Journal of Substance Use*, 15(1):31–41.

Gmel G et al. (2005). Drinking patterns and traffic casualties in Switzerland: matching survey data and police records to design preventive action. *Public Health*, 5:426–436.

Graham K et al. (2006). Bad nights or bad bars? Multi-level analysis of environmental predictors of aggression in late-night large-capacity bars and clubs. *Addiction*, 101(11): 1569–1580.

Graham K, Homel R (2008). *Raising the bar: preventing aggression in and around bars, pubs and clubs*. Cullompton, Willan Publishing.

Grubesic TH, Pridemore WA (2011). Alcohol outlets and clusters of violence. *International Journal of Health Geographics*, 10:30.

Hughes K et al. (2008). Alcohol, nightlife and violence: the relative contributions of drinking before and during nights out to negative health and criminal justice outcomes. *Addiction*, 103(1):60–65.

Hughes K et al. (2011a). Drinking behaviours and blood alcohol concentration in four European drinking environments: a cross-sectional study. *BMC Public Health*, 11(1):918.

Hughes K et al. (2011b). Environmental factors in drinking venues and alcohol-related harm: the evidence base for European intervention. *Addiction*, 106(S1):37–46.

Johnsson KO, Berglund M (2003). Education of key personnel in student pubs leads to a decrease in alcohol consumption among the patrons: a randomized controlled trial. *Addiction*, 98(5):627–633.

Johnsson KO, Berglund M (2009). Do responsible beverage service programs reduce breath alcohol concentration among patrons: a five-month follow-up or a randomized controlled trial. *Substance Use & Misuse*, 44:1592–1601.

Jones L, Hughes K, Atkinson AM (2011). Reducing harm in drinking environments: a systematic review of effective approaches. *Health & Place*, 17(2):508–518.

Ker K, Chinnock P (2008). Interventions in the alcohol server setting for preventing injuries. *Cochrane Database of Systematic Reviews*, (3):CD005244.

Livingston M, Chikritzhs T, Room R (2007). Changing the density of alcohol outlets to reduce alcohol-related problems. *Drug and Alcohol Review*, 26:557–66.

Miller P et al. (2011). Do community interventions targeting licensed venues reduce alcohol-related emergency department presentations? *Drug and Alcohol Review*, 30:546–553.

Rabinovich L et al. (2009). *The affordability of alcohol beverages in the European Union: understanding the link between alcohol affordability, consumption and harms*. Cambridge, RAND Europe.

Rabinovich L et al. (2011). *Draft final report: further study on the affordability of alcoholic beverages in the EU.* Cambridge, RAND Europe.

Rammohan V et al. (2011). Effects of dram shop liability and enhanced overservice law enforcement initiatives on excessive alcohol consumption and related harms. *American Journal of Preventive Medicine*, 41(3):334–343.

Ricci G et al. (2008). Prevalence of alcohol and drugs in urine of patients involved in road accidents. *Journal of Preventive Medicine and Hygiene*, 49(2):89–95.

Rowe SC et al. (2010). Establishments licensed to serve alcohol and their contribution to police-recorded crime in Australia: further opportunities for harm reduction. *Journal of Studies on Alcohol and Drugs*, 71(6):909–916.

Toomey TL et al. (2008). A randomized trial to evaluate a management training program to prevent illegal alcohol sales. *Addiction*, 103(3):405–413.

Wahl S, Kriston L, Berner M (2010). Drinking before going out – a predictor of negative nightlife experiences in a German inner city area. *International Journal of Drug Policy*, 21(3):251–254.

Warpenius K, Holmila M, Mustonen H (2010). Effects of a community intervention to reduce the serving of alcohol to intoxicated patrons. *Addiction*, 105:1032–1040.

WHO Regional Office for Europe (2009). *Evidence for the effectiveness and cost–effectiveness of interventions to reduce alcohol-related harm.* Copenhagen, WHO Regional Office for Europe (http://www.euro.who.int/__data/assets/pdf_file/0020/43319/E92823.pdf, accessed 12 February 2012).

Alcohol and the workplace

Peter Anderson

Introduction

The workplace provides several opportunities for implementing prevention strategies to reduce the harm done by alcohol, since the majority of adults are employed and spend a significant proportion of their time at work. The workplace can also be a risk factor for harmful alcohol use. Many studies have found significant associations between stress in the workplace and elevated levels of alcohol consumption, an increased risk of problem drinking and alcohol dependence.

Evidence has found that alcohol, and in particular heavy drinking, increases the risk of unemployment and, for those in work, absenteeism. Alcohol, especially episodic heavy drinking, has also been found to increase the risk of arriving late at work and leaving early or disciplinary suspension, resulting in loss of productivity; a higher turnover due to premature death; disciplinary problems or low productivity from the use of alcohol; inappropriate behaviour (such as behaviour resulting in disciplinary procedures); theft and other crime; poor co-worker relations and low company morale. Studies suggest that alcohol consumption may have more effect on productivity on the job than on the number of workdays missed. Overall, the costs of lost productivity feature as the dominant element in studies of the social costs arising from the harm done by alcohol, being about half of the total social cost of alcohol in the EU.

Despite the evidence of the negative impact of alcohol on the workplace, there are surprisingly few good-quality scientific studies to inform policy and practice, and of those that have been undertaken, it is not always possible to conclude convincingly the best approaches. Increasingly, and as an alternative, evidence suggests that prevention activities at the workplace to reduce the harm done by alcohol should be embedded in broader workplace health promotion and well-being at work initiatives.

This chapter summarizes a review of workplace-based policies (Anderson, 2012) undertaken for the European Workplace Alcohol project financed by the EU (European Workplace Alcohol project, 2012) which, in turn, was informed by a review (Anderson, 2010) within the EU-financed FASE project (FASE, 2012). The review of the European Workplace Alcohol project provided the background for the Scientific Opinion of the Science Group of the European Alcohol and Health Forum on Alcohol, Work and Productivity (European Commission, 2011).

Alcohol and employment

Impaired productivity

There are three lines of evidence to suggest that alcohol could impair productivity: its impact on the accumulation of human capital through education; the time in life when alcohol leads to ill health and premature death; and its importance in the working age population, relative to other risk factors, in leading to impaired health and premature death.

There is evidence, although not from all studies (Dee & Evans, 2003), that drinking (Koch & Ribar, 2001), in particular binge-drinking (Renna, 2009), has an impact on the number of years at school (Lye & Hirschberg, 2010). Other studies find a significant negative relationship between drinking and measures of education that reflect the quality of human capital accumulation (Wolaver, 2007). Carrell, Hoekstra & West (2011) exploited the discontinuity in drinking at age 21 years at the United States Air Force Academy, where the minimum legal drinking age is strictly enforced. They found that drinking caused significant reductions in academic performance, particularly for the highest-performing students. Their results indicated that the negative consequences of alcohol consumption extended beyond the narrow segment of the population at risk of more severe, low-frequency, outcomes.

Globally, the peak age of alcohol-related death is in middle age and older middle age, a time often of peak performance at work (Rehm, Taylor & Room, 2006). As an illustration of this, the age of alcohol-related hospitalizations and deaths has been estimated in the United Kingdom for conditions solely and partially due to alcohol (Jones et al., 2008). For both men and women, the estimated highest absolute number of deaths from alcohol-attributable conditions occurred in the age ranges 45–64 years, an important part of the working age population (OECD, 2010). On the other hand, it can be seen for both men and women that young people, although having a small absolute number of alcohol-related deaths, have the highest proportion of all deaths due to alcohol-related conditions in the age group. This is not surprising, since the highest rates of heavy alcohol use and binge-drinking occur among young adults aged 18–25 years. In 2010, youth unemployment in developed countries and the EU stood at over 18% (ILO, 2011). This is a risk factor for alcohol-related harm. In addition, for those joining the labour market, the transition from school to the labour force represents a high-risk time for alcohol use. Specific job-related influences associated with problem drinking, including job stressors and participation in work-based drinking networks, may pose a particular problem for young adults as they attempt to fit into their new workplace (Bray et al., 2011).

Looking globally at the age range 25–59 years, the age group in the EU with the highest employment rates (OECD, 2010), alcohol use is the world's number one risk factor for ill health and premature death (expressed as DALYs) (WHO, 2011). Lost productivity costs feature as the dominant element in studies of social costs arising from the harm done by alcohol (Rehm et al., 2006; Collins & Lapsley, 2008; Saar, 2009; Rehm et al., 2009).

Recession, unemployment and alcohol

Many commentators have expressed concern that the present economic downturn is adversely affecting public health as a result of job losses, contributing to mental health or addiction problems and the adoption of less healthy lifestyles. If this is the case, it is important to know how better to mitigate the impact of the economic downturn and how to improve the reintegration of unemployed people with mental health or addiction problems into the labour market (Litchfield, 2011).

Becoming unemployed does seem to worsen alcohol-related harm. An analysis of the effect of economic downturns in the EU undertaken by Stuckler et al. (2009) found that a more than 3% increase in unemployment was associated with an increase in suicide rates at ages younger than 65 years (4.45% increase; 95% CI: 0.65–8.24; 250–3220 potential excess deaths [mean 1740] EU-wide) and an increase in deaths from "alcohol abuse" (28.0% increase; 95% CI: 12.30–43.70; 1550–5490 potential excess deaths [mean 3500] EU-wide). Unemployment seems to lead to less alcohol consumed but to more risky patterns of drinking (Dee, 2001). Stuckler et al. (2009) found that for every US$ 10 higher investment in active labour market programmes, there was a 0.04% lower effect of a 1% rise in unemployment on suicide rates in people younger than 65 years. When the spending was greater than US$ 190 per head per year (adjusted for PPP), rises in unemployment would have no adverse effect on suicide rates. The associations between US$ 100 rises in income, social welfare spending and health care spending per capita (PPP in US$ for 2000) on cause-specific mortality in 15 EU countries for the period 1980–2005 have been studied by Stuckler, Basu & McKee (2010). Increases in social spending in areas other than health care were significantly associated with reductions in alcohol-related mortality. For every US$ 100 rise in social welfare spending excluding health care, alcohol-related mortality fell by 2.8%.

Only a limited number of studies have tried to estimate the role of alcohol in unemployment, but they do suggest that heavy drinking increases the risk of unemployment. A meta-analysis of papers that studied the relationship between alcohol consumption and earnings suggested that there was a lack of labour force participation by individuals who consume large amounts of alcohol (Lye & Hirschberg, 2010).

Absenteeism

A Swedish study found that a one-litre increase in total consumption was found to be associated with a 13% increase in sickness absence among men ($p < 0.05$) but not among women (Norström, 2006). In Norway, a similar study found that a one-litre increase in total alcohol consumption was associated with a 13% increase in sickness absence among men, but the effect of alcohol was not significant among women (Norstrom & Moan, 2009).

Micro-level data from Finland and Sweden have shown that alcohol consumption and alcohol-related problems are usually (Upmark et al., 1997; Upmark, Moller & Romelsjo, 1999; Johansson, Bockerman & Uutela, 2008; Laaksonen et al., 2009; Salonsalmi et al., 2009), but not always (Hensing, Holmgren & Mårdby, 2011) positively associated with the number of sickness absence days and disability pensions for both men and women. A large study of 13 582 Australian workers found clear evidence for the impact of drinking patterns on absenteeism (Roche et al., 2008). Compared to low-risk drinkers, workers drinking at short-term high-risk levels (110 g alcohol or more on any one day for a man and 70 g alcohol or more on any one day for a woman) at least yearly, at least monthly or at least weekly were 3.1, 8.7 and 21.9 times, respectively, more likely to report alcohol-related absenteeism.

Presenteeism

Currently, there is no universal agreement on the most appropriate method for measuring or monetizing presenteeism (when employees come to work ill and perform below par due to illness) or suboptimal performance at work (Schultz, Chen & Edington, 2009; Chen et al., 2008). It is typically measured as the costs associated with reduced work output, errors on the job or failure to meet company production standards. Despite the measurement difficulties, a range of studies have stressed the importance of health risk factors, including alcohol, in increasing presenteeism (Cooper & Dewe, 2008; Schultz Chen & Edington, 2009; Goetzel et al., 2004).

An Australian study of 78 000 workers found that drug and alcohol use disorders increased the risk of presenteeism 2.6-fold, and 8.6-fold, when compounded with psychological distress (Holden et al., 2011).

Alcohol and earnings

When compared with abstainers, some studies have found a positive effect of alcohol on wages, a wage premium from light drinking (Peters, 2004; van Ours, 2004; Lee, 2003; Barrett, 2002). It seems, however, that part of this effect is due to misclassification and the specific problem of combining former drinkers, who might have increased health problems and thus lower wages, and long-term abstainers into one pooled group of abstainers, called the "former drinker error" (Jarl, Gerdtham & Selin, 2009). A meta-analysis of 11 studies that have reported a positive impact of alcohol consumption on earnings (a proxy measure of productivity) suggested that the relationship was an artefact, with alcohol consumption proving to be an imperfect proxy for all personality traits that have a positive influence on human capital (Lye & Hirschberg, 2010).

Alcohol and people other than the drinker

Almost all studies that have estimated the social costs of alcohol have not estimated the costs of alcohol borne by people other than the drinker. Given the impact of alcohol on people other than the drinker, this seems a rather important omission. One study has estimated the social costs of alcohol borne by people other than the drinker – an Australian study which reviewed the magnitude and range of harm from alcohol to others (Laslett et al., 2010) – and found its impact on productivity to be important. The total cost of harm from people other than the drinker was Australian $14.2 billion. Of this, A$ 9.3 billion resulted from lost productivity costs due to lost and wasted time because of the activities of a heavy drinker, while A$ 801 million was due to direct work-related costs split between extra hours worked (A$ 453 million) and absenteeism (A$ 348 million). The annual cost of extra hours worked by workers because of a co-worker's drinking (A$ 453 million) is comparable with estimates of absenteeism due to one's own drinking (A$ 3 68 million, Collins & Lapsley, 2008). Overall, it was found that the inclusion of harm done by alcohol to people other than the drinker, after deducting any double-counting, doubled the social costs from A$ 12.2 billion to A$ 23.5 billion.

Adverse work environment

Analysis of the Whitehall II occupational cohort of London-based civil servants study found that there was a clear grade gradient for women, with those in the highest two grades having the highest proportion of problem drinkers, which was not the case for men (Head, Stansfeld & Siegrist, 2004). In men, the effort–reward imbalance was associated with alcohol dependence after taking account of age and employment grade, with those classified as putting in high efforts but receiving low rewards having the highest risk of being alcohol-dependent. This association was also seen for women, although it was not as marked. In addition, a low decision latitude in women was associated with increased risk of alcohol dependence. Neither high job demands nor low work support were associated with alcohol dependence. These associations between work characteristics and alcohol dependence did not appear to be mediated through physical illness, poor mental health, or adverse changes in social supports or network size.

The workplace could influence workers and those who do not drink in three other ways: (i) through the perceived physical availability of alcohol at work, including the ease of obtaining it at work and of using it during working hours and breaks; (ii) through descriptive norms or the extent to which members of an individual's workplace social network use alcohol or work while impaired by alcohol at work; and (iii) through injunctive norms or the extent to which members of an individual's workplace social network approve of using or working under the influence of alcohol at work. A study of employees in the United States found that injunctive norms predicted alcohol use and impairment, and descriptive norms predicted alcohol use before and during work as well as workplace impairment (Frone & Brown, 2010). Another study of abstinent employees in the United States found that all three dimensions of the workplace substance use climate were negatively related to workplace safety, positively related to work strain, and negatively related to employees' morale (Frone, 2009). A study in the United States revealed that employees who were problem drinkers were more likely than non-problem drinkers to perceive lower levels of certain workplace alcohol social controls against drinking. Employees who were problem-drinkers were also found to be more likely than abstainers and non-problem-drinkers to report higher levels of certain forms of social availability of alcohol at the workplace (Berger, 2009). In Canada, workplace alcohol availability predicted general alcohol problems (Hodgins, Williams & Munro, 2009). In another set of studies of the impact of alcohol use by colleagues among municipal employees, Bennett et al. (2004) found that the presence of a drinking climate correlated with job stress and job withdrawal more than did reports of individual colleagues' drinking. The drinking climate and individual job stress were negatively associated with cohesion of the work group. A drinking climate combined with low cohesion resulted in increased vulnerability for job stress, job withdrawal, health problems and performance (work accidents and absences). Moreover, work group cohesion appeared to attenuate the negative impact of exposure to drinking norms. Increased vulnerability was exacerbated in employees with higher proportions of jobs involving risk, such as machine work.

Despite the structural relationships between the work environment and the risk of alcohol use disorders, few intervention studies have investigated the impact of changing work structures on reducing workplace alcohol-related harm (Roman & Blum 1996; 2002). An exception to this is a study that compared two work settings with distinctly different managerial cultures (Ames, Grube & Moore, 2000). One setting had a traditional hierarchical United States management design and the other was based on a Japanese management model transplanted to the United States. Although overall alcohol consumption rates in both populations were similar, the traditional management design was associated with more permissive norms regarding drinking before or during work shifts (including breaks) and higher workplace drinking rates. By contrast, the transplant management design was associated with greater enforcement of alcohol policies which, in turn, predicted more conservative drinking norms and lower alcohol availability at work. Qualitative research clearly indicated that the transplant design facilitated the social control of alcohol problems, whereas the traditional design appeared to undermine such control.

The workplace can also act as a role model for families and communities. The vast majority of European adults in the EU are in full-time employment. They are also parents and members of social networks. The workplace is also a site for young people for job experience and internships. Thus, what goes on in the workplace (such as workplace alcohol-free environments) can, through social networks of families and friends, have an impact outside the workplace. For example, data from the Framingham heart study shows that alcohol consumption behaviour spreads in social networks up to three degrees of separation (Rosenquist et al., 2010), with a dose–response relationship between the fraction of a principal's friends and family who drank heavily or abstained at one examination and the average number of drinks per day that the principal reported at the next examination. Being surrounded by heavy drinkers increased the reported alcohol consumption by about 70% (CI: 35–142%) compared with those who were not connected to any heavy drinkers. Conversely, being surrounded by abstainers decreased reported alcohol consumption by half. Each additional heavy drinker increased the likelihood that a principal drank heavily by 18% (CI: 11–25%) and decreased the likelihood that a principal abstained by 7% (CI: 2–12%). Conversely, each additional abstainer significantly reduced the likelihood that a principal drank heavily by 10% (CI: 4–15%) and increased the likelihood that a principal abstained by 22% (CI: 17–28%).

A number of analyses have found that occupations with the highest alcohol-related death rates are bar staff, seafarers and publicans and those working in the catering, entertainment and hospitality industries, as well as those working in the construction industries (Coggon et al.,

2009; 2010; Hemmingsson et al., 1997). Interestingly, while male medical practitioners were among the occupations with the highest alcohol-related mortality in the 1960s to 1980s in the United Kingdom (England and Wales), they were among the occupations with the lowest alcohol-related mortality in 2001–2005 (Romeri, Baker & Griffiths, 2007).

Workplace interventions

A systematic review of workplace interventions for alcohol-related problems (Webb et al., 2009) identified only 10 intervention studies, of which 5 were counselling-based interventions, 4 were mail-out/feedback/brief intervention studies and 1 was a peer support programme. Counselling and related interventions comprised three broad types of strategy: psychosocial skills training; brief intervention, including feedback of results of self-reported drinking, lifestyle factors and general health checks; and alcohol education delivered via an internet web site. The psychosocial interventions included peer referral, team-building and stress management and skills derived from the social learning model. For health checks, topics covered in addition to alcohol were smoking, exercise, diet, weight, stress, depression, blood pressure, cholesterol, diabetes, cancer, safety and preventive health-care risks. The counselling-based interventions either reported no effect (Hermansson et al., 1998) or the effect was small, self-reported only, or measured desire to change rather than actual behaviour (Bennett et al., 2004; Heirich & Sieck, 2000; Cook, Back & Trudeau, 1996; Lapham, Gregory & McMillan, 2003). The four mail-out/feedback/brief intervention studies (Anderson & Larimer, 2002; Richmond et al., 2000; Matano et al., 2007; Walters & Woodall, 2003) were practical and possibly sustainable interventions that achieved outcomes somewhat comparable to the more intensive counselling interventions. The outcomes were, however, self-reported.

An additional study published since the systematic review of Webb et al. (2009) of screening and brief intervention for risky alcohol consumption at the workplace in the transport sector failed to find evidence of effect (Hermansson et al., 2010). An employee assistance office-based programme compared the impact of a brief intervention for at-risk drinking compared with usual care. At three month follow-up, employees who received the brief intervention had significantly reduced their presenteeism (but not absenteeism), with costs saved from improved productivity over the four-week period prior to the three-month assessment of US$ 1200 per employee over the usual care group (Osilla et al., 2009). Consistent with other experience, the increase in productivity came primarily from increases in presenteeism and not decreases in absenteeism (Goetzel et al., 2009).

Peer support programmes

One of the 10 studies identified by Webb et al. (2009) used objective outcome measures to describe the impact of a workplace peer-focused substance abuse programme in the transportation industry implemented in phases from 1988 to 1990 (Spicer & Miller, 2005; Miller, Zaloshnja & Spicer, 2007). The programme focused on changing workplace attitudes towards on-the-job substance use in addition to training workers to recognize and intervene with colleagues who have a problem. The programme was strengthened by federally mandated random drug- and alcohol-testing (implemented, respectively, in 1990 and 1994). With time-series analysis, the association of monthly injury rates and costs with the phased programme implementation were analysed, controlling for same industry injury trend. The combination of the peer-based programme and testing was associated with an approximate one third reduction in the injury rate, avoiding an estimated US$ 48 million in the employer's costs in 1999. That year, the peer-based programme cost the company US$ 35 and testing cost another US$ 35 per employee. The programme avoided an estimated US$ 1850 in the employer's injury costs per employee in 1999, corresponding to a benefit–cost ratio of 26:1. In another study of urban transit workers, perceived co-worker support was found to attenuate the link between frequency of heavy episodic drinking and absenteeism (Bacharach, Bamberger & Biron, 2010).

Computer-delivered programmes

A meta-analysis of 75 randomized clinical trials that have included more than 35 000 participants and evaluated 82 separate computer-delivered health promotion interventions concluded that computer-delivered interventions can help individuals to make improvements in various forms of health behaviour including substance and alcohol use (11 studies) (Portnoy et al., 2008). A greater intervention dose strengthened the impact on reduction of substance use. One study has evaluated the efficacy of an alcohol web-based personalized feedback programme delivered in the workplace to young adults (Doumas & Hannah, 2008). Results indicated that participants in the intervention group reported significantly lower levels of drinking than those in the control group at 30-day follow-up. This was particularly true for participants classified as high-risk drinkers at the baseline assessment. Adding a 15-minute motivational interviewing session did not increase the efficacy of the web-based feedback programme.

Mandatory screening

A Cochrane systematic review to assess the effect of alcohol and drug mandatory screening of occupational drivers in preventing injury or work-related effects, such as sickness absence related to injury (Cashman et al., 2009), identified only two interrupted time-series studies (Swena, 1999; Spicer & Miller, 2005). Spicer & Miller reported the evaluation of the workplace peer-focused substance abuse prevention and early intervention programme (entitled PeerCare) implemented against the background of federally mandated random drug- and alcohol-testing in an interrupted time-series design from 1983 to 1996. Swena reported the evaluation of federally mandated random drug-testing on countrywide fatal truck accidents in an interrupted time-series design from 1983 to 1997. The workplace-based study in the transport company found that while alcohol testing was associated with a decrease in the level of injuries immediately following the intervention (-1.25 injuries/100 person years; 95% CI: -2.29 – -0.21), there was no significant change in the already long-term downward trend (-0.28 injuries/100 person years/year; 95% CI: -0.78–0.21). For federally mandated random drug-testing, both studies found no immediate beneficial effect but did find significant declines in the yearly injury rate additional to the existing downward trend over time: -0.19 injuries/100 person years/year; 95% CI: -0.30 – -0.07 for the transport company (Spicer & Miller, 2005), and -0.83 fatal accidents/100 million vehicle miles/year; 95% CI: -1.08 – -0.58 for the countrywide study (Swena, 1999).

A systematic review of interventions for preventing injuries in the construction industry only identified five studies (van der Molen et al., 2007), one of which evaluated whether or not drug-free workplace programmes, which included alcohol, prevented occupational injuries (Wickizer et al., 2004). Overall, in the construction, manufacturing and service industries, companies with drug-free workplace programmes had a net reduction of 3.33 injuries per 100 person/years, compared with companies without drug-free workplace programmes, with the reduction being greater in the service than in the construction and manufacturing industries.

Embedding alcohol programmes within health promotion programmes

Interventions that focus on health promotion and on different lifestyles rather than on the disease have shown higher participation as well as greater improvement in drinking risk than those focusing on punitive sanctions (Sieck & Heirich, 2010). An inclusive model of prevention minimizes the likelihood that employees will feel singled out for their alcohol use or their participation in an intervention programme in a punitive context. The evidence for the impact of health promotion programmes at the workplace is, however, limited. In a systematic review, Kuoppala, Lamminpaa & Husman (2008) identified 46 studies which suggested that workplace health promotion could improve work ability (risk ratio (RR) 1.4; range 1.2–1.7) although not decrease sickness absences. Overall, there was no impact on mental or physical well-being. Exercise programmes were effective in increasing overall well-being (RR 1.25; range 1.05–1.47) and work ability (RR 1.38; range 1.15–1.66), but education and psychological methods were not. In another systematic review of 27 identified papers, Kuoppala and colleagues (2008) found evidence that leadership at work can improve job well-being (RR 1.40, range 1.36–1.57) and decrease sick leave (RR 0.73, range 0.70–0.89) and disability pensions (RR 0.46, range 0.42–0.59).

A systematic review of the effects of workplace health promotion programmes on presenteeism identified 14 studies, of which 10 were described as presenting preliminary evidence of promising effects on presenteeism in their respective employee populations and work settings (Cancelliere et al., 2011). Two studies were described as showing the strongest evidence, one of which involved worksite exercise (Nurminen et al., 2002) and the second, the impact of a supervisor education programme regarding mental health promotion (Takao et al., 2006). However, even in these two studies, the evidence is either not present or very weak. In the study by Nurminen et al. (2002), women engaged in physically demanding laundry work were individually randomized into an intervention or control group, with the intervention subjects participating in worksite exercise training guided by a physiotherapist. The women were followed up at 3, 8, 12 and 15 months. Although at 12 months, the number of workers with perceived good work ability increased more in the intervention group than in the control group (11.0%, 95% CI: 0.2–21.9), as did the health-related prognosis of work ability at 8 months (8.1%, 95% CI: 0.5–16.3), there were no statistically significant differences between the two groups as regards job satisfaction, work ability index or sick leaves.

In a programme to reduce work-related stress in a sake brewery, Nishiuchi et al. (2007) found that although an education programme for stress reduction could improve supervisors' knowledge about stress reduction in the workplace, it had no impact on their attitudes or behaviour. Not surprisingly, then, the job stress education programme for supervisors on psychological distress and job performance among their immediate subordinates made no difference to psychological distress or job performance among male and female subordinates (Takao et al., 2006, the study referred to above as showing an impact). The only exception to this was among the 27 young male subordinates in white collar occupations, for whom there was some evidence for improvement in stress reduction and job performance. Nevertheless, independent of the programme, subordinates working under supervisors with good listening attitudes and skills reported slightly (but statistically significant) better job control and less stress than those subordinates working under supervisors with poor listening attitudes and skills (Mineyama et al., 2007).

Workplace wellness programmes

Despite the limited evidence for effective workplace health promotion programmes, some meta-analyses have reported positive returns on investment for workplace wellness programmes (Chapman, 2003; 2005; Baicker, Cutler & Song, 2010). In their systematic review of United States-based studies, Baicker and colleagues (2010) identified 22 studies reporting on employees' health care costs and 22 on absenteeism costs. It should be remembered that in the

United States, over 60% of Americans get their health care insurance through an employment-based plan. By far the most frequently used method of workplace intervention delivery was the health risk assessment, a survey that gathers baseline self-reported health data from the employee, which are in turn used by the employer to tailor the subsequent intervention. The second most common wellness intervention mechanism was the provision of self-help education materials, individual counselling with health care professionals or on-site group activities led by trained personnel. The use of incentives to motivate participation was seen in 30% of programmes. The most common foci of the programmes were obesity and smoking. Seventy-five per cent of programmes focused on more than one risk factor, including stress management, back care, nutrition, alcohol consumption, blood pressure and preventive care, in addition to smoking and obesity. Medical costs were found to fall US$ 3.27 for every dollar spent on wellness programmes, and absentee day costs fall by US$ 2.73 for every dollar spent. Of course, there are some caveats to the validity of the findings: first, the firms implementing wellness programmes are likely to be those with the highest expected returns; second, it is difficult to gauge the extent of publication bias, with programmes seeing a high return on investment most likely to be published; third, almost all of the studies were implemented by large employers, who are more likely than others to have the resources and economies of scale necessary both to implement and to achieve broad savings through employee wellness programmes; and, fourth for the topic of this report, we have no idea how much, if any, the positive effects are alcohol-specific.

Conclusions for policy and practice

Well-being at work initiatives

Given the lack of a robust evidence base for workplace-based approaches that focus on individual counselling, it may be better to focus activities under the umbrella of well-being at work initiatives (Robertson & Cooper, 2011), particularly those that focus on presenteeism (Cancelliere et al., 2011), and those that bring a good return on investment (Baicker, Cutler & Song, 2010). The core factors that promote well-being at work include structural factors (Podsakoff, LePine & LePine, 2007) and management and leadership styles (Yarker, Lewis & Donaldson-Feilder, 2008), all of which could make an impact on alcohol-related harm.

Alcohol-free workplaces

Many workplaces are already alcohol-free. Increasing the extent of alcohol-free workplaces will result in reductions in alcohol-related workplace accidents and injuries, as well as creating a culture for a more healthy relationship with alcohol that has an impact on families and friends through social networks.

Occupational target groups

Based on the rates of alcohol-related mortality, three target groups stand out for action: those working in the retail alcohol trade, labourers in the construction industry, and seafarers and dockers. The example of English doctors who, over the course of 20–30 years fell in the occupational league table of alcohol-related mortality from near the top to near the bottom, demonstrates that change can be made. The behaviour of doctors has been taken as a marker of how harmful lifestyle forms of behaviour are perceived in a country.

Population target groups

Although this might be interpreted as covering everyone, there are in fact two target groups, the young and the older middle age: the young, because they suffer from both differential high rates of unemployment and risky drinking, compounded by the stresses when joining the labour market, and the middle-aged, because they have the absolute highest rates of alcohol-related disability and premature death. The United States-based multisite initiative on substance use prevention programmes for young adults in the workplace provides, for example, a frame for action for young people, which has been commonly neglected in the past (Bray, Galvin & Cluff, 2011).

References

Ames GM, Grube JW, Moore RS (2000). Social control and workplace drinking norms: a comparison of two organizational cultures. *Journal of Studies on Alcohol,* 61(2):203–219.

Anderson BK, Larimer ME (2002). Problem drinking and the workplace: an individualized approach to prevention. *Psychology of Addictive Behaviors,* 16:243–251.

Anderson P (2010). *A report on the impact of workplace policies and programmes to reduce the harm done by alcohol to the economy.* Utrecht, National Institute for Alcohol Policy (http://www.faseproject.eu/wwwfaseprojecteu/fase-elements/literature-study-workplace.htm, accessed 24 February 2012).

Anderson P (2012). *Alcohol and the workplace.* Barcelona, Department of Health, Government of Catalonia.

Bacharach SB, Bamberger P, Biron M (2010). Alcohol consumption and workplace absenteeism: the moderating effect of social support. *Journal of Applied Psychology*; 95(2):334–348.

Baicker K, Cutler D, Song Z (2010). Workplace wellness programs can generate savings. *Health Affairs,* 29(2):304–111.

Barrett G (2002). The effect of alcohol consumption on earnings. *Economic Record*, 78:79–96.

Bennett JB et al. (2004). Team awareness, problem drinking, and drinking climate: workplace social health promotion in a policy context. *American Journal of Health Promotion,* 19:103–113

Berger LK (2009). Employee drinking practices and their relationships to workplace alcohol social control and social availability. *Journal of Workplace Behavioral Health,* 24:367–382.

Bray JW, Galvin DM, Cluff LA, eds. (2011). *Young adults in the workplace: a multisite initiative of substance use prevention programs.* Research Triangle Park, NC, RTI Press (http://www.rti.org/pubs/bk-0005-1103-cluff.pdf, accessed 14 February 2012).

Cancelliere C et al. (2011). Are workplace health promotion programs effective at improving presenteeism in workers? A systematic review and best evidence synthesis of the literature. *BMC Public Health,* 11:395.

Carrell SE, Hoekstra M, West JE (2011). Does drinking impair college performance? Evidence from a regression discontinuity approach. *Journal of Public Economics,* 95(1–2):54–62.

Cashman CM et al. (2009). Alcohol and drug screening of occupational drivers for preventing injury. *Cochrane Database of Systematic Reviews,* (2):CD006566.

Chapman LS (2003). Meta-evaluation of worksite health promotion economic return studies. *The Art of Health Promotion,* 6:1–16.

Chapman LS (2005). Meta-evaluation of worksite health promotion economic return studies: 2005 update. *American Journal of Health Promotion,* 19:1–11.

Chen H et al. (2008). Assessing productivity loss and activity impairment in severe or difficult-to-treat asthma. *Value Health,* 11(2):231–239.

Coggon D et al. (2010). Occupation and mortality related to alcohol, drugs and sexual habits. *Occupational Medicine,* 60:348–353.

Coggon D et al. (2009). *Occupational mortality in England and Wales, 1991–2000*. London, Office for National Statistics.

Collins DJ, Lapsley HM (2008). *The costs of tobacco, alcohol and illicit drug abuse to Australian society in 2004/05*.Canberra, Commonwealth of Australia (National Drug Strategy Monograph, No. 64).

Cook RF, Back AS, Trudeau J (1996). Preventing alcohol use problems among blue-collar workers: a field test of the Working People program. *Substance Use and Misuse*, 31(3):255–275.

Cooper C, Dewe P (2008). Well-being – absenteeism, presenteeism, costs and challenges. *Occupational Medicine*, 58:522–524.

Dee TS (2001). Alcohol abuse and economic conditions: evidence from repeated cross-sections of individual-level data. *Health Economics,* 10:257–270.

Dee TS, Evans W (2003). Teen drinking and educational attainment: evidence from two-sample instrumental variables estimates. *Journal of Labor Economics,* 21:178–209.

Doumas DM, Hannah E (2008). Preventing high-risk drinking in youth in the workplace: a web-based normative feedback program. *Journal of Substance Abuse Treatment,* 32:263–271.

European Commission (2011). *Alcohol, work and productivity. Scientific Opinion of the Science Group of the European Alcohol and Health Forum*. Brussels, European Commission (http://ec.europa.eu/health/alcohol/docs/science_02_en.pdf, accessed 21 February 2012).

European Workplace Alcohol project [web site] (2012). Barcelona, Department of Health of the Government of Catalonia (http://www.eurocare.org/eu_projects/ewa, accessed 21 February 2012).

FASE (2012). Focus on Alcohol Safe Environment (FASE) [web site]. Utrecht, Dutch Institute for Alcohol Policy (http://www.faseproject.eu/wwwfaseprojecteu/about-fase/, accessed 21 February 2012).

Frone MR (2009). Does permissive workplace substance use climate affect employees who do not use alcohol and drugs at work? A U.S. national study. *Psychology of Addictive Behavior,* 23:386–390.

Frone MR, Brown AL (2010). Workplace substance-use norms as predictors of employee substance use and impairment: a survey of U.S. workers. *Journal of Studies on Alcohol and Drugs,* 71:526–534.

Goetzel RZ et al. (2004). Health, absence, disability, and presenteeism cost estimates of certain physical and mental health condition affecting U.S. employers. *Journal of Occupational and Environmental Medicine,* 46(4):398–412.

Goetzel RZ et al. (2009). The relationship between modifiable health risk factors and medical expenditures, absenteeism, short-term disability, and presenteeism among employees at Novartis. *Journal of Occupational and Environmental Medicine,* 51(4):487–499.

Head J, Stansfeld SA, Siegrist J (2004). The psychosocial work environment and alcohol dependence: a prospective study. *Journal of Occupational and Environmental Medicine,* 61:219-224.

Heirich M, Sieck CJ (2000). Worksite cardiovascular wellness programs as a route to substance abuse prevention. *Journal of Occupational and Environmental Medicine,* 42:47–56.

Hemmingsson T et al. (1997). Alcoholism in social classes and occupations in Sweden. *International Journal of Epidemiology,* 26:584–591.

Hensing G, Holmgren K, Mårdby AC (2011). Harmful alcohol habits were no more common in a sample of newly sick-listed Swedish women and men compared with a random population sample. Alcohol and *Alcoholism*, 46(4): 471–477.

Hermansson U et al. (1998). Feasibility of brief intervention in the workplace for the detection and treatment of excessive alcohol consumption. *International Journal of Occupational and Environmental Health,* 4:71–78.

Hermansson U et al. (2010). Screening and brief intervention for risky alcohol consumption in the workplace: results of a 1-year randomized controlled study. *Alcohol and Alcoholism,* 45:252–257.

Hodgins DC, Williams R, Munro G (2009). Workplace responsibility, stress, alcohol availability and norms as predictors of alcohol consumption-related problems among employed workers. *Substance Use & Misuse,* 44:2062–2079.

Holden L et al. (2011). Health-related productivity losses increase when the health condition is co-morbid with psychological distress: findings from a large cross-sectional sample of working Australians. *BMC Public Health,* 11:417–426.

ILO (2011). *Global employment trends 2011: the challenge of a jobs recovery.* Geneva, International Labour Office.

Jarl J, Gerdtham UG, Selin KH (2009). Medical net cost of low alcohol consumption – a cause to reconsider improved health as the link between alcohol and wage? *Cost Effectiveness and Resource Allocation,* 7:17.

Johansson E, Bockerman P, Uutela A (2008). Alcohol consumption and sickness absence: evidence from microdata. *European Journal of Public Health,* 19(1):19–22.

Jones L et al. (2008). *Alcohol-attributable fraction for England. Alcohol-attributable mortality and hospital admissions.* Liverpool, John Moores University, Northwest Public Health Observatory (http://www.nwph.net/nwpho/Publications/AlcoholAttributableFractions.pdf, accessed 14 February 2012).

Koch S, Ribar D (2001). A siblings analysis of the effects of alcohol consumption onset on educational attainment. *Contemporary Economic Policy,* 19:162–174.

Kuoppala J, Lamminpaa A, Husman P (2008). Work health promotion, job wellbeing, and sickness absences – a systematic review and meta-analysis. *Journal of Occupational and Environmental Medicine,* 50(11):1216–1227.

Kuoppala J et al. (2008). Leadership, job well-being, and health effects – a systematic review and a meta-analysis. *Journal of Occupational and Environmental Medicine,* 50(8):904–915.

Laaksonen M et al. (2009). Health-related behaviours and sickness absence from work. *Occupational and Environmental Medicine,* 66:840–847.

Lapham SC, Gregory C, McMillan G (2003). Impact of an alcohol misuse intervention for health care workers.1. Frequency of binge drinking and desire to reduce alcohol use. *Alcohol and Alcoholism,* 38:176–182.

Laslett AM et al. (2010). *The range and magnitude of alcohol's harm to others.* Fitzroy, VIC, AER Centre for Alcohol Policy Research, Turning Point Alcohol and Drug Centre, Eastern Health.

Lee Y (2003). Wage effects of drinking in Australia. *Australian Economic Review,* 36:265–282.

Litchfield P (2011). Mitigating the impact of an economic downturn on mental well-being. In: Robertson I, Cooper C, eds. *Well-being. Productivity and happiness at work.* Basingstoke, Palgrave Macmillan.

Lye J, Hirschberg J (2010). Alcohol consumption and human capital: a retrospective study of the literature. *Journal of Economic Surveys,* 24(2): 309–338.

Matano RA et al. (2007). A pilot study of an interactive web site in the workplace for reducing alcohol consumption. *Journal of Substance Abuse Treatment,* 32:71–80.

Miller TR, Zaloshnja E, Spicer RS (2007). Effectiveness and benefit-cost of peer-based workplace substance abuse prevention. *Accident analysis and prevention,* 39(3):565–573.

Mineyama S et al. (2007). Supervisors' attitudes and skills for active listening with regard to working conditions and psychological stress reactions among subordinate workers. *Journal of Occupational Health,* 49:81–87.

Nishiuchi K et al. (2007). Effects of an education program for stress reduction on supervisor knowledge, attitudes and behaviour in the workplace: a randomized controlled trial. *Journal of Occupational Health,* 49:190–198.

Norstrom T (2006). Per capita alcohol consumption and sickness absence. *Addiction,* 110:1421–1427.

Norstrom T, Moan IS (2009). Per capita alcohol consumption and sickness absence in Norway. *European Journal of Public Health,* 16(4):383–388.

Nurminen E et al. (2002). Effectiveness of a worksite exercise program with respect to perceived work ability and sick leaves among women with physical work. *Scandinavian Journal of Work, Environment & Health,* 28(2):85–93.

OECD (2010). *OECD factbook (2010): Economic, environmental and social statistics.* Paris, Organisation for Economic Co-operation and Development.

Osilla KC et al. (2009). Exploring productivity outcomes from a brief intervention for at-risk drinking in an employee assistance program. *Addictive Behaviors,* 35:194–200.

Peters BL (2004). Is there a wage bonus from drinking? Unobserved heterogeneity examined. *Applied Economics,* 36:2299–2315.

Podsakoff NP, LePine JA, LePine MA (2007). Differential challenge stressor–hindrance stressor relationships with job attitudes, turnover intentions, turnover, and withdrawal behavior: a meta-analysis. *Journal of Applied Psychology,* 92(2):438–454.

Portnoy DB et al. (2008). Computer-delivered interventions for health promotion and behavioral risk reduction: a meta-analysis of 75 randomized controlled trials, 1988–2007. *Preventive Medicine,* 47(1):3–16.

Rehm J et al. (2006). *The costs of substance abuse in Canada 2002.* Ottawa, ON, Canadian Centre on Substance Abuse.

Rehm J et al. (2009). Global burden of disease and injury and economic cost attributable to alcohol use and alcohol use disorders. *Lancet,* 373(9682):2223–2233.

Rehm J, Taylor B, Room R (2006). Global burden of disease from alcohol, illicit drugs and tobacco. *Drug and Alcohol Review,* 25:503–513.

Renna F (2009). Alcohol abuse, alcoholism, and labor market outcomes: looking for the missing link. *Industrial & Labor Relations Review,* 62(1):92–103.

Richmond R et al. (2000). Evaluation of a workplace brief intervention for excessive alcohol consumption: the Workscreen Project. *Preventive Medicine,* 30:51–63.

Robertson I, Cooper C (2011). *Well-being. Productivity and happiness at work.* Basingstoke, Palgrave Macmillan.

Roche AM et al. (2008). Workers' drinking patterns: the impact on absenteeism in the Australian workplace. *Addiction,* 103:738–748.

Roman PM, Blum TC (1996). Alcohol: a review of the impact of worksite interventions on health and behavioral outcomes. *American Journal of Health Promotion,* 11:135–149.

Roman PM, Blum TC (2002). The workplace and alcohol problems prevention. *Alcohol Research and Health,* 26(1):49–57.

Romeri E, Baker A, Griffiths C (2007). Alcohol-related deaths by occupation, England and Wales, 2001–05. *Health Statistics Quarterly,* 35:6–12.

Rosenquist JN et al. (2010). The spread of alcohol consumption behaviour in a large social network. *Annals of Internal Medicine,* 152:426–433.

Saar I (2009). The social costs of alcohol misuse in Estonia. *European Addiction Research,* 15(1):56–62.

Salonsalmi A et al. (2009). Drinking habits and sickness absence: the contribution of working conditions. *Scandinavian Journal of Public Health,* 37:846–854.

Schultz AB, Chen CY, Edington DW (2009). The cost and impact of health conditions on presenteeism to employers: a review of the literature. *Pharmacoeconomics,* 27(5):365–378.

Sieck CJ, Heirich M (2010). Focusing attention on substance abuse in the workplace: a comparison of three workplace interventions. *Journal of Workplace Behavioral Health,* 25:72–87.

Spicer RS, Miller TR (2005). Impact of a workplace peer-focused substance abuse prevention and early intervention program. *Alcoholism: Clinical and Experimental Research*, 29(4):609–611.

Stuckler D, Basu S, McKee M (2010). Budget crises, health, and social welfare programmes. *British Medical Journal*, 341:77–79.

Stuckler D et al. (2009). The public health effect of economic crises and alternative policy responses in Europe: an empirical analysis. *Lancet*, 374:315–323.

Swena DD (1999). Effect of random drug screening on fatal commercial truck accident rates. *International Journal of Drug Testing*, 2:1–13.

Takao S et al. (2006). Effects of the job stress education for supervisors on psychological distress and job performance among their immediate subordinates: a supervisor-based randomized controlled trial. *Journal of Occupational Health,* 48(6):494–503.

Upmark M et al. (1997). Predictors of disability pension among young men. *European Journal of Public Health,* 1:20–28.

Upmark M, Moller J, Romelsjo A (1999). Longitudinal, population-based study of self-reported alcohol habits, high levels of sickness absence and disability pensions. *Journal of Epidemiology and Community Health,* 53:223–229.

van der Molen H et al. (2007). Interventions for preventing injuries in the construction industry. *Cochrane Database of Systematic Reviews*, (4) CD006251.

van Ours J (2004). A pint a day raises a man's pay; but smoking blows that gain away. *Journal of Health Economics,* 23:863–886.

Walters ST, Woodall W (2003). Mailed feedback reduces consumption among moderate drinkers who are employed. *Prevention Science,* 4:287–294.

Webb G et al. (2009). A systematic review of work-place interventions for alcohol-related problems. *Addiction,* 104:365–377.

WHO (2011). *Global status report on alcohol and health.* Geneva, World Health Organization.

Wickizer TM et al. (2004). Do drug-free workplace programs prevent occupational injuries? Evidence from Washington State. *Health Services Research*, 39(1):91–110.

Wolaver A (2007). Does drinking affect grades more for women? Gender differences in the effects of heavy episodic drinking in college. *The American Economist*, 51:72–88.

Yarker J, Lewis R, Donaldson-Feilder E (2008). *Management competencies for preventing and reducing stress at work*. London, Health and Safety Executive.

Availability of alcohol

Esa Österberg

Introduction

The physical availability of alcoholic beverages refers to the ease or convenience of obtaining alcohol for drinking purposes. Regulations on physical availability include the monopolization or licensing of on- or off-premise retail sales of alcoholic beverages as well as general or special limits on opening times for retail alcohol sales. Physical availability also includes regulations covering the location of alcohol retail sale outlets, special on- or off-premise sales practices (such as over the counter or self-service sales), and rules on the maximum size or number of drinks to be served to customers at one time. These regulations can also dictate who is allowed to purchase alcoholic beverages in licensed premises or off-premises. Usually these regulations concern the legal age limits for selling, buying, possessing or drinking alcoholic beverages and refusing the sale of alcoholic beverages to intoxicated persons or even to certain religious or ethnic groups (Room et al., 2002). There can also be rules relating to the rationing of alcohol sales which may be specified according to age and sex. Sometimes the physical availability of alcoholic beverages has been converted to economic availability by mention of the effective or full price of alcoholic beverages (see, for example, Chaloupka, Grossman & Saffer, 2002; Babor et al., 2010, and the chapter on pricing of alcohol).

Historical evaluations show that total bans on alcohol production and sales can reduce alcohol-related harm. However, where there has been a substantial demand for alcohol, it has been met during prohibition by an informal market often organized by criminal operators. Independently of the research evidence of the effects of total bans on alcohol consumption and related harm, total prohibition is clearly politically not an acceptable alternative in contemporary Europe (Anderson & Baumberg, 2006).

A licence issued by the local or central administration is required in many countries before alcoholic beverages can be sold. For off-premise retail sales, where alcoholic beverages are consumed elsewhere than in the place of purchase, regulations can be made on the type, strength and packaging of the beverages that can be sold as well as the times and places for the sale of alcoholic beverages. For on-premise sales, where alcohol is consumed in the point of sale, regulations can also specify drink sizes or require the staff to receive training in responsible service of beverages. When the licensing system is used to restrict the number of outlets, most often the aim is to prevent harm and public disorder by limiting the supply of alcohol. These kinds of regulation, as well as restrictions on the number of outlets for alcoholic beverages, have been shown to have an effect on alcohol consumption and related harm. Some studies have also indicated that changing either the hours or days of alcohol sales can affect alcohol-related harms (Anderson & Baumberg, 2006).

There is consistent evidence that government monopolies on off-premise retail sales of alcoholic beverages affect alcohol consumption and related harm to both young people and adults. When Finland allowed the sale of medium beer (alcohol content at most 4.7%) in grocery stores in 1969, total alcohol consumption rose nearly 50% in a year (Mäkelä, Österberg & Sulkunen, 1981; Mäkelä, 2002). When medium strength beer could be bought in grocery stores in Sweden between 1965 and 1977, total alcohol consumption was some 15% higher than before 1965 or after 1977 (Noval & Nilsson, 1984; Tiihonen, 2011). From 1915 on, beer sales were prohibited in Iceland. When retail sales of beer in alcohol monopoly liquor stores and licensed restaurants were allowed in March 1989, its consumption rose considerably. In both Finland and Sweden, these changes in beer consumption did not bring down the consumption of other beverage categories, but in Iceland the increased availability of beer did shift consumption from distilled spirits to beer (Olafsdottir, 1998; 2002; Mäkelä, 2002; Noval & Nilsson, 1984).

About half a century ago, broad restrictions on who could purchase alcoholic beverages were fairly common. The most extensive of such systems was the Bratt rationing scheme in Sweden in force until 1955, which assigned a quantitatively defined upper limit for spirits purchases per person with different rations for males and females and for younger age groups. Studies have shown that rationing systems in Greenland, Poland and Sweden reduced alcohol-related harm (Anderson & Baumberg, 2006). In Spitzbergen (Norway) there still exists a rationing system for purchases of alcoholic beverages.

Legal minimum age limits are widely practised availability restrictions targeted to young people, although limits vary from country to country, ranging typically from 16 to 21 years of age (Anderson & Baumberg, 2006). A review of 132 studies published between 1960 and 2000 found strong evidence that changes in laws for minimum drinking ages can have substantial effects on drinking by young people and alcohol-related harm. These effects often lasted well after the young people reached the legal drinking age (Wagenaar & Toomey, 2002). A study from Denmark, where a minimum age limit of 15 years was introduced for off-premise purchases in 1998, found that drinking by young people above as well as below the age limit was affected (Møller, 2002). There were no age limits on off-premise alcohol sales in Denmark from 1970 to July 1998 (Karlsson & Österberg, 2002). Recent innovative work has also examined the long-term effects of minimum limits on the drinking age (Gruenewald, 2011).

According to the material collected in the AMPHORA project, in at least four EU member states the legal age limits have been raised during the last decade, namely Denmark in 2004 and 2011, France in 2009, Malta in 2009 and Belgium in 2009. No EU member state has lowered the legal age limits for alcoholic beverages in the last four decades.

The full benefits of legal drinking-age limits are only realized if these limits are effectively enforced. Despite laws on the minimum drinking age, young people have often been able to buy alcoholic beverages. In most of the countries participating in the European School Survey Project on Alcohol and Other drugs (ESPAD) in 2003, most schoolchildren aged 15–16 years thought that getting any type of alcoholic beverage was fairly or very easy, rising to 70–95% for beer and wine (Hibell et al., 2004). Even moderate increases in enforcement can reduce sales to minors by as much as 35–40%, especially when combined with media and other community activities (Wagenaar & Toomey, 2002).

In the European Comparative Alcohol Study (ECAS) looking at alcohol control in EU member states and Norway in 1995, it was noted that between 1950 and 2000, some ECAS countries with no age limits in the 1950s began to implement legal age limits for buying alcoholic beverages, and in some ECAS countries age limits were raised. In Finland and Sweden, however, the age limits were lowered (Österberg & Karlsson, 2002). In 2000 there were still some ECAS countries with no legal age limits for at least some categories of alcoholic beverage in off-premise sales.

New research regarding the effects of changes in legal age limits has concentrated on the effectiveness of policies related to enforcement and support for a minimum legal drinking age. In Europe, the growing interest in enforcing minimum legal restrictions on the drinking age is connected to the increased use of test purchasing (mystery shoppers) as a way to check how retail traders are following the relevant laws. In Finland and Sweden, the off-premise retail alcohol monopoly companies hire independent test purchasers to check how well the monopoly's employees are following the rules requiring the presentation of an identification card. In Finland and Sweden, all customers looking younger than 25 years of age have to present an identity card, even though it is legal in these countries to sell distilled spirits to customers aged 20 years (Vihmo & Österberg, 2011).[5]

As well as the alcohol monopoly companies, nongovernmental organizations, especially those concerned with young people, have been active in mystery shopping. There are also community-based research projects, such as the Finnish PAKKA project, which use trial purchasers (Holmila, Karlsson & Warpenius, 2010). Trial purchasers hired by the monopoly companies or in the PAKKA project are young-looking people who have reached the legal purchase age. Some nongovernmental organizations in the Nordic countries are in fact using trial purchasers who actually are under age, which can lead to legal problems.

Test purchasing is being used more and more in the continental European countries and the British Isles (Gosselt et al., 2007; Tael, 2011). In these countries, trial purchasers are usually hired by state or local authorities as well as by nongovernmental organizations in order to check to what extent underage people are able to buy alcoholic beverages and to put pressure on retailers to improve their enforcement of the legal age limits.

Underage alcohol use is also linked to access through informal family and social networks. According to the ESPAD study, in many countries the most common sources of alcoholic beverages among underage drinkers are parents, siblings and friends (Hibell & Skretting, 2009; Paschal, Grube & Kypri, 2009).

Ratings of measures controlling physical availability of alcohol

There is not much new research evidence from EU member states regarding controls on the availability of alcoholic beverages since the report *Alcohol in Europe. A public health perspective* was published in 2006. Denmark and Lithuania changed their shop opening laws in 2010, leading to an increase in alcohol availability, whereas Estonia and Ireland introduced stricter rules regarding alcohol sales times in 2008, as did Finland and Italy in 2007. These changes have not, however, been studied, partly because the changes in availability have been quite small.

The second edition of *Alcohol: no ordinary commodity*, published in 2010, gives the latest situation on the physical availability of alcohol by rating policy options by their effectiveness, breadth of research support and cross-national testing (Babor et al., 2010; see also WHO Regional Office for Europe, 2009). Babor and his colleagues give all interventions affecting the physical availability of alcohol at least two pluses out of three for effectiveness, research support and cross-national testing (Table 9). The WHO publication *Evidence for the effectiveness and cost–effectiveness of interventions to reduce alcohol-related harm* summarizes the evidence relating to physical availability, and finds that there is consistent evidence that alcohol-related

---

[5] In Sweden, 20 years for all alcoholic beverages; in Finland, 20 years for spirits and 18 years for wine and beer.

harm can be reduced by maintaining or raising the minimum purchasing age for alcohol, introducing government monopolies on the retail sale of alcoholic beverages, and regulating and limiting the density of outlets as well as times for alcohol sale (WHO Regional Office for Europe, 2009).

Table 9. Ratings of strategies and interventions affecting physical availability of alcoholic beverages

Strategy or intervention	Effectiveness[a]	Research support[b]	Cross-national testing[c]
Ban on sales	+++	+++	++
Minimum legal purchase age	+++	+++	++
Rationing	++	++	++
Government monopoly of retail sales	++	+++	++
Restrictions on times of sale	++	++	+++
Restrictions on density of outlets	++	+++	++
Different availability by alcohol strength	++	+++	++

[a] The likely impact of interventions reflecting the strength of scientific evidence establishing whether a particular strategy is effective in reducing alcohol consumption and/or alcohol-related problems: + evidence of limited effectiveness; ++ evidence of moderate effectiveness; +++ evidence for a high degree of effectiveness.
[b] Research support goes beyond the quality of science to look at the quantity and consistency of the available evidence, including conflicting evidence: + one or two well-designed studies have been undertaken; ++ several studies have been completed, sometimes in different countries but no integrative reviews were available; +++ enough studies have been completed to permit integrative literature reviews or meta-analyses.
[c] Evidence for an intervention drawn from studies conducted in different countries, regions, subgroups and social classes: + strategy studied in at least two countries, ++ in several countries, +++ in many countries.

Source: Babor et al, 2010.

A systematic review (Hahn et al., 2010) concluded that there was sufficient evidence to show that increasing alcohol sales times by two or more hours increases alcohol-related harm. Although the review did not find sufficient evidence for the impacts of smaller increases in sales hours, a new study in Norway examining changes in bar closing times in 18 cities has since found that each one-hour extension to bar opening hours was associated with a significant increase in assaults (Rossow & Norstrom, 2011). With the international trend towards increased bar opening hours, few studies have examined the impacts of reduced alcohol service hours in bars. However, in Newcastle, Australia, pub closing times were restricted in 2008 following police and public complaints about violence, disorderly behaviour and property damage related to intoxication.[6] A study associated the restrictions with a relative reduction in recorded assaults of 37% (Kypri et al., 2010).

A systematic review assessed the effectiveness of limiting the density of alcohol outlets so as to reduce excessive alcohol use and related harms (Bryden et al., 2011). Again, the trend towards increased alcohol liberalization meant that it found few studies assessing the impact of restricting the density of outlets. However, most studies identified showed greater alcohol outlet density to be associated with increased alcohol consumption and harms, including injury, violence, crime and medical harm. A range of new studies have added weight to this evidence, associating higher densities of licensed premises with alcohol-related harm, particularly violence (Grubesic & Pridemore, 2011; Livingston, 2011a; Connor et al., 2011; Livingston, 2011b).

---

[6] The restrictions covered 14 pubs. Opening times were restricted to between 0500 and 0300 hours, with an 0100 lock-in that prevented new customers entering after that time. However, a legal challenge by the pubs led to the restrictions being amended to 0330 closing and 0130 lock-in after the first four months.

Conclusions for policy and practice

The accumulation of research evidence about the impact of interventions regarding the physical availability of alcohol has been really impressive during recent decades. Much more is known now of the effects of restrictions on the physical availability of alcohol than half a century ago when *Alcohol control policies in public health perspectives* was published in 1975. According to Babor and his colleagues (2010), among the 10 best practices (besides alcohol taxes) in preventive alcohol policies are interventions in the physical availability of alcohol such as the minimum purchase age, government alcohol monopolies, and restrictions on the times of sale and the density of outlets selling alcoholic beverages.

References

Anderson P, Baumberg B (2006). *Alcohol in Europe. A public health perspective*. London, Institute of Alcohol Studies.

Babor TF et al. (2010). *Alcohol: no ordinary commodity. Research and public policy,* 2nd ed. Oxford, Oxford University Press.

Bryden A et al. (2012). A systematic review of the influence on alcohol use of community level availability and marketing of alcohol. *Health and Place*, 18(2):349–357.

Chaloupka FJ, Grossman M, Saffer H (2002). The effects of price on alcohol consumption and alcohol-related problems. *Alcohol Research and Health,* 26:22–34.

Connor JL et al. (2011). Alcohol outlet density, levels of drinking and alcohol-related harm in New Zealand: a national study. *Journal of Epidemiology and Community Health*, 65(10): 841–846.

Gosselt JF et al. (2007). Mystery shopping and alcohol sales: do supermarkets and liquor stores sell alcohol to underage customers? *Journal of Adolescent Health*, 41:302–308.

Grubesic TH, Pridemore WA (2011). Alcohol outlets and clusters of violence. *International Journal of Health Geographics*, 10:30.

Gruenewald PJ et al. (2006). Alcohol prices, beverage quality and the demand for alcohol: quality substitutions and price elasticities. *Alcoholism: Clinical and Experimental Research*, 30:96–105.

Hahn RA et al. (2010). Effectiveness of policies restricting hours of alcohol sales in preventing excessive alcohol consumption and related harms. *American Journal of Preventive Medicine*, 39(6):590–604.

Hibell B et al. (2004). *The ESPAD report 2003: alcohol and other drug use among students in 35 European countries.* Stockholm, Swedish Council for Information on Alcohol and Other Drugs and the Pompidou Group at the Council of Europe.

Hibell B, Skretting A (2009). *The 2007 ESPAD report: substance use among students in 35 European countries.* Stockholm, The Swedish Council for Information on Alcohol and Other Drugs.

Holmila M, Karlsson T, Warpenius K (2010). Controlling teenagers' drinking: effects of a community-based prevention project. *Journal of Substance Use,* 15:201–214.

Karlsson T, Österberg E (2002). Denmark. In: Österberg E, Karlsson T, eds. *Alcohol policies in EU member states and Norway. A collection of country reports*. Helsinki, Stakes:120–139.

Kypri K et al. (2010). Effects of restricting pub closing times on night-time assaults in an Australian city. *Addiction*, 106:303–310.

Livingston M (2011a). Alcohol outlet density and harm: comparing the impacts on violence and chronic harms. *Drug and Alcohol Review*, 30(5):515–523.

Livingston M (2011b). A longitudinal analysis of alcohol outlet density and domestic violence. *Addiction*, 106(5):919–925.

Mäkelä K, Österberg E, Sulkunen P (1981). Drink in Finland: increasing alcohol availability in a monopoly state. In: Single E, Morgan P, deLint J, eds. *Alcohol, society and state II: the social history of control policy in seven countries*. Toronto, Addiction Research Foundation:31–59.

Mäkelä P (2002). Who started to drink more? A reanalysis of the change resulting from a new alcohol law in Finland in 1969. In: Room R, ed. *The effects of Nordic alcohol policies: analyses of changes in control systems*. Helsinki, Nordic Council for Alcohol and Drug Research:71–82.

Møller L (2002). Legal restrictions resulted in a reduction of alcohol consumption among young people in Denmark. In: Room R, ed. *The effects of Nordic alcohol policies: analyses of changes in control systems*. Helsinki, Nordic Council for Alcohol and Drug Research:155–166.

Noval S, Nilsson T (1984). Mellanölets effect på konsumtionsnivån och tillväxten hos den totala alkoholkonsumtionen [The effects of medium beer on consumption levels and the rise in overall alcohol consumption]. In: Nilsson T, ed. *När mellanölet försvann [When the beer disappeared]*. Linköping, Linköping University:77–93.

Olafsdottir H (1998). The dynamics in shifts in alcoholic beverage preference: effects of the legalization of beer in Iceland. *Journal of Studies on Alcohol,* 59:107–114.

Olafsdottir H (2002). Legalizing beer in Iceland. In: Room R, ed. *The effects of Nordic alcohol policies: analyses of changes in control systems*. Helsinki, Nordic Council for Alcohol and Drug Research:95–116.

Österberg E, Karlsson T (2002). Alcohol policies in EU member states and Norway in the second half of the twentieth century. In: Österberg E, Karlsson T, eds. *Alcohol policies in EU member states and Norway. A collection of country reports*. Helsinki, Stakes:433–460.

Paschall MJ, Grube JW, Kypri K (2009). Alcohol control policies and alcohol consumption by youth: a multi national study. *Addiction*, 104:1849–1855.

Room R et al. (2002). *Alcohol in developing societies: a public health approach*. Helsinki, Finnish Foundation for Alcohol Studies.

Rossow I, Norstrom T (2011). The impact of small changes in bar closing hours on violence. The Norwegian experience from 18 cities. *Addiction*, 107(3):530–537.

Tael M (2011). *Alkohoolsete jookide testostemise pilooturing [Pilot study on alcohol purchase by youngsters]*. Tallinn, National Institute for Health Development.

Tiihonen J et al. (2011). *Päivittäistavarakaupoisssa myytävien juomien alkoholipitoisuuden alentamisen vaikutus alkoholin kulutukseen ja kuolemiin [The effects of decreasing the upper alcohol content limit of alcoholic beverages permitted to be sold in grocery stores]*. Helsinki, Government Institute for Economic Research.

Vihmo J, Österberg E (2011). *Information on the Nordic alcohol market 2011*. Helsinki, Alko.

Wagenaar AC, Toomey TL (2002). Effects of minimum drinking age laws: review and analyses of the literature from 1960 to 2000. *Journal of Studies on Alcohol,* 63:S206–225.

WHO Regional Office for Europe (2009). *Evidence for the effectiveness and cost–effectiveness of interventions to reduce alcohol-related harm*. Copenhagen, WHO Regional Office for Europe (http://www.euro.who.int/__data/assets/pdf_file/0020/43319/E92823.pdf, accessed 12 February 2012).

The impact of alcohol marketing

Avalon de Bruijn

Introduction

The manufacturers of alcoholic beverages market their products in various ways to encourage consumption of their products. The marketing of alcoholic beverages is a multifaceted, strategic and long-term endeavour which starts with product development and innovation and uses commercial communications to extol the benefits of, and remove barriers to, consumption (Fig.17).

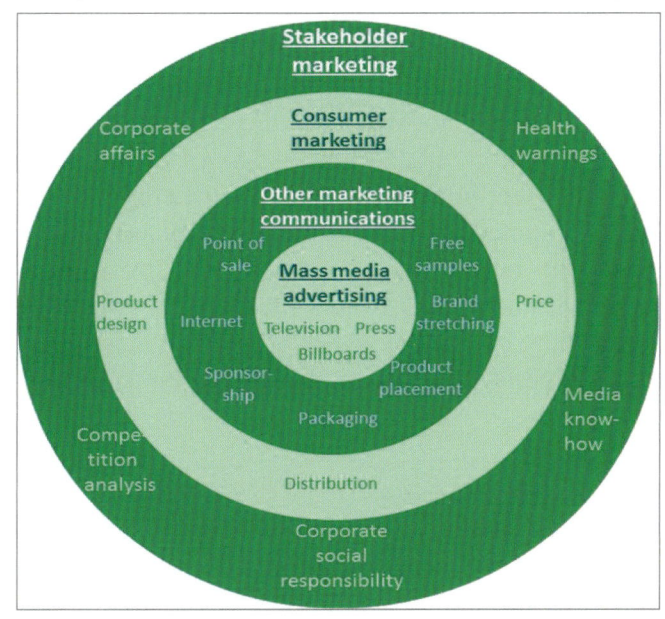

Fig. 17. The multifaceted character of marketing

Source: Hastings et al., 2010.

Research suggests that exposure to tobacco marketing increases smoking by adolescents (Wellman et al., 2006; DiFranza et al., 2006; Paynter & Edwards, 2009; Lovato et al., 2003) and exposing young people to food marketing increases their food intake and the likelihood of obesity (Hastings et al., 2003; Harris et al., 2009; Nestle, 2006). It has been debated whether there is also a causal relationship between exposure to alcohol marketing and young people's drinking. In science there is a long discourse on this topic.

Population-based studies from the 1980s and 1990s mostly examined the relationship between United States data on changes in per capita consumption (generally measured by alcohol sales figures) and changes in levels of alcohol advertising (generally measured by data on advertising expenditure) (Anderson & Baumberg, 2006). The studies show mixed results: most show little or no effect of alcohol advertising on overall consumption. Later studies using similar approaches have found significant effects of alcohol advertising on the consumption of alcohol and on alcohol-related problems (Saffer, 1991; Saffer & Dave, 2004).

A meta-analysis of 132 econometric studies found a small but significant positive association between alcohol advertising and alcohol consumption, although only for spirits advertising (Gallet, 2007). Looking at alcohol advertising expenditure data across the United States, Saffer & Dave (2006) found, when controlling for alcohol price, income and a number of sociodemographic variables, that advertising expenditure had an independent yet modest effect on the monthly number of adolescents drinking and binge-drinking. It was estimated that a 28% reduction in alcohol advertising would reduce the monthly share of adolescent drinkers from 25% to between 24% and 21%. For binge-drinking, the reduction would be from 12% to between 11% and 8%. Controlling for price, income and minimum legal drinking age across the United States, Nelson (2003) found that although total alcohol consumption was negatively related to a ban on the advertising of spirit prices (the ban led to less consumption, coefficient -0.009), it was positively related to a ban on billboards (which accounted for only 8% of total alcohol advertising) which led to more consumption, coefficient 0.054. In a more recent study, the effect of partial bans was reported not to have affected alcohol consumption in 17 countries over 26 years (Nelson, 2010). A systematic review of 10 studies concluded that variations in the use of advertising restrictions and the methodological challenges meant that findings were inclusive and any positive effects were likely to be modest at most (Booth et al., 2008).

Methodological challenges in econometric studies have been discussed by Anderson & Baumberg (2006). In most econometric studies, alcohol advertising expenditure is used as an approximate measure of the effectiveness of alcohol marketing. These expenditure data are often limited to traditional media spending and exclude significant components, such as "below the line" promotions, sponsorship or the use of viral advertising where consumers pass marketing messages to each other. As econometric studies measure the effectiveness of alcohol advertising only in terms of spending, they do not distinguish between less or more attractive content in the advertisements, although advertising essentially works by creating positive expectancies and beliefs about the product.

Another approach consists in studying the effects of exposure to alcohol advertising on drinking patterns. Small effects between exposure to alcohol advertising and the likelihood of adolescents drinking were found in early surveys, but owing to cross-sectional designs these studies were not able to establish causality (Anderson & Baumberg, 2006).

In 1998, the National Institute on Alcohol Abuse and Alcoholism (NIAAA) funded three longitudinal studies that followed thousands of American adolescents for several years. Although mixed results were found on the impact of televised alcohol advertising, the studies generally suggest that exposure to alcohol marketing is a significant predictor of drinking behaviour among adolescents. Through their prospective design and the innovative approaches used to measure the exposure to alcohol marketing, these studies contributed significantly to the evidence base (Gordon, Hastings & Moodie, 2010).

More longitudinal studies have since been carried out (Box 3). For example, a study by Collins et al. (2007) found that 12-year-olds who are highly exposed to overall alcohol advertising are more likely to start drinking a year later, compared to 12-year-olds who are only slightly exposed to alcohol advertising. A longitudinal study by Pasch et al. (2007) found that the exposure of sixth graders (aged 10–12 years) to outdoor alcohol advertisements was associated with subsequent intentions to drink alcohol.

Advertising for alcoholic beverages in the mass media may be the most noticeable form of alcohol marketing but it represents only part of the big picture (Fig. 17). "Below the line"

> **Box 3. Some examples from longitudinal studies of long-term effects of exposure to alcohol advertising on drinking behaviour.**
>
> - 12-year-olds who are highly exposed to overall alcohol advertising (75th percentile) are 50% more likely to start drinking a year later compared to 12-year-olds who are slightly exposed to alcohol advertising (25th percentile) (Collins et al., 2007).
>
> - Youngsters who watch 60% more alcohol advertisements on television than average are 44% more likely to have ever used beer, 34% more likely to have ever used wine/hard liquor and 26% more likely to have ever drunk three or more drinks on one occasion (Stacy et al., 2004).
>
> - In non-drinking 13-year-olds, exposure to in-store beer displays predicts the age of onset of drinking (Ellickson et al., 2005).
>
> - Non-drinking 12-year- olds who possess a promotional item from an alcohol producer, or would like to have one, have a 77% higher chance of drinking one year later compared to children who do not possess a promotional item and do not have a favourite alcohol brand (McClure et al., 2009).
>
> - Teenage boys who own an alcohol-branded promotional item are 1.78 times more likely to start using alcohol than boys who do not own such items. For girls, the figure was 1.74 (Fisher et al., 2007).
>
> - Teenagers who are highly exposed to alcohol advertising will drink more alcohol when they are in their twenties. In youngsters who have been slightly exposed to alcohol advertising, alcohol consumption stabilizes in the early twenties (Snyder et al., 2006).

marketing, such as point-of-sale promotions or merchandising, the use of other products connected with alcohol brands, sponsorship, or alcohol advertising in online media have only recently received research attention.

Hurtz et al. (2007) found in a cross-sectional study that youngsters aged 11–14 years who were regularly exposed to point-of-sale alcohol advertising in grocery stores were more likely to start drinking than those not so exposed.

Fisher et al. (2007) and McClure et al. (2006; 2009) found that ownership of alcohol-branded promotional items influenced young people's drinking behaviour. Controlling for a broad range of confounding variables, both the possession of a promotional item and an attitudinal susceptibility towards alcohol brands predicted the age of onset of drinking as well as binge-drinking among 10–14-year-olds (McClure et al., 2006; McClure et al., 2009). Henriksen et al. (2008) found that non-drinking 12-year-olds who possess an alcohol-branded promotional item, or would like to have one, have a 77% higher chance of drinking one year later compared to children who are not similarly sensitive to alcohol marketing.

The impact of sports sponsorship by alcohol manufacturers is largely unexplored. O'Brien et al. (2011) examined the relationship between direct alcohol sponsorship and drinking in adult sports people in Australia. Hazardous drinking (as measured by the Alcohol Use Disorders Identification Test) was more common among those receiving some form of alcohol-related support than among those who reported no alcohol sponsorship.

Gordon et al. (2010) and Gordon, MacKintosh & Moodie (2011) in the UK examined the influence of exposure of 12–14-year-olds to a wide range of alcohol marketing, including marketing in the new media. After controlling for confounding variables, involvement with alcohol marketing at baseline was predictive of both uptake of drinking and increased frequency of drinking at follow-up two years later (Gordon, MacKintosh & Moodie, 2011).

The impact of product placement, for example in broadcast entertainment programming, is another un-researched area. The portrayal of alcohol is, however, common in television programming and films, with or without linkage to product placement, and such portrayals provide a programming context which may influence drinking behaviour as such or may interact with embedded alcohol commercials.

Sargent et al. (2006) examined the impact of exposure to alcohol portrayal in films over time, a method copied by Hanewinkel et al. (2009) and Morgenstern et al. (2011). The prospective studies conducted in Germany and the United States drew similar conclusions: the start of alcohol use was positively related to baseline exposure to alcohol advertising.

Immediate effects

Experimental studies have been conducted to examine the short-term effects of alcohol advertising on drinking behaviour (see Box 4). The findings indicate that seeing alcohol cues on the screen (either in films or commercials) directly influences the actual drinking behaviour of adolescents (Engels et al., 2009). It is hypothesized that this has to do with the more or less unconscious process of imitation of what is seen on the screen: if the main character in a film is portrayed drinking alcohol, the viewer unconsciously "imitates" and takes a sip as well (Koordeman et al., 2011a; Koordeman et al., 2011b). An imitation effect was not consistently found among all experimental groups but it was visible among those who were already familiar with drinking larger quantities of alcohol. More research is needed to provide greater insight into the short-term effects of alcohol on different groups, for example women versus men or light drinkers versus heavy drinkers.

> **Box 4. Examples of experimental study findings on short-term effects of exposure to alcohol advertising**
>
> - Young men who watched a film which included many portrayals of alcohol (*American Pie 2*), interrupted by alcohol commercials, consumed twice as much alcohol during the viewing than young men who saw a more "neutral" film (*40 days and 40 nights*) interrupted by neutral commercials (Engels et al., 2009).
> - Young men who watched the original version of the film *What happens in Vegas*, including alcohol, drank almost twice as much alcohol as men who watch a censored version of the same film, in which the alcohol slots had been removed (Koordeman et al., 2011a).
> - Regular alcohol users (>7 glasses per week) drank 2.5 times more alcohol in the cinema after seeing several alcohol commercials preceding the film (*Watchmen*) compared with regular alcohol users who saw several neutral commercials (Koordeman, Anschutz & Engels, 2009). This effect was not found for the participants with a relatively low alcohol use (<7 glasses per week).

The long-term and immediate effects of alcohol marketing are summarized in Table 10.

The EU has financed a number of projects on marketing (Annex 4).

Conclusions for policy and practice

Since the publication of the report *Alcohol in Europe* (Anderson & Baumberg, 2006), the evidence base relating to the impact of alcohol marketing has grown considerably, supporting the conclusion that alcohol marketing affects young people's drinking behaviour. It has been found that exposure to alcohol marketing increases the likelihood that young people start to drink alcohol, and that among young people who have started to use alcohol, such exposure increases

Table 10. Summary of evidence on the impact of alcohol marketing published since 2006

Effects	Key studies	Key findings
Long-term effect of alcohol advertising in mass media	Anderson et al. (2009); Babor et al. (2010); Smith & Foxcroft (2009); WHO (2009).	Although studies of the impact of televised alcohol advertising on adolescents' drinking behaviour show mixed results, longitudinal studies show a general impact of alcohol advertising in the mass media on adolescents' drinking behaviour.
Long-term effects of non-media alcohol marketing	McClure et al. (2006); McClure et al. (2009); Gordon, MacKintosh & Moodie (2011); Hanewinkel & Sargent (2009), Morgenstern et al. (2011), Sargent et al. (2006).	The impact of sponsorship, viral marketing and marketing in digital media is an understudied area. Longitudinal studies of non-media alcohol marketing show an impact of alcohol marketing on drinking behaviour.
Immediate effect of alcohol advertising	Engels et al. (2009); Koordeman, Anschutz & Engels (2009); Koordeman et al. (2011a); Koordeman et al. (2011b).	First experimental studies suggest a direct effect of exposure to alcohol marketing cues (in films and/or television commercials) on the drinking behaviour of adolescents. More research is needed to give insight on differences in effects in sub-groups (for example, gender, or light versus heavy drinkers).

the frequency of drinking and the amount of alcohol consumed. The size of the effect demonstrated in the studies, while statistically significant, tends to be relatively small. The studies measuring exposure to alcohol marketing usually focus on selected channels and forms of marketing, and do not grasp the cumulative nature of overall marketing influences (see Fig. 17).

The impact of alcohol marketing through non-media channels, or through new channels such as the internet, has only recently begun to be addressed in research. Together with experimental studies and longitudinal studies carried out in Europe, such studies will shed further light on the cumulative effects of exposure to alcohol advertising through multiple marketing channels, and on mechanisms that explain the impact of alcohol marketing.

In view of the impact of alcohol marketing on the drinking behaviour of young people, effective regulation of alcohol marketing can contribute substantially to reducing alcohol-related harm by delaying the onset of drinking and by lessening the incentives to drink more. Regulations can be mandated by law, established by a sector or by individual companies through voluntary codes of responsible conduct, or set by a combination where legislation creates the framework for self-regulation. Irrespective of the approach, the key issue is to establish a regulatory framework that incorporates monitoring and enforcement and is able to tackle the cross-national nature of alcohol marketing (Babor et al., 2010).

In 2009, the Science Group of the European Alcohol and Health Forum concluded:

> Based on the consistency of findings across the studies, the confounders controlled for, the dose response relationships, as well as the theoretical plausibility and experimental findings regarding the impact of media exposure and commercial communications, it can be concluded from the studies reviewed that alcohol marketing increases the likelihood that adolescents will start to use alcohol, and to drink more if they are already using alcohol.

References

Anderson P, Baumberg B (2006). *Alcohol in Europe. A public health perspective*. London, Institute of Alcohol Studies.

Anderson P et al. (2009). Impact of alcohol advertising and media exposure on adolescent alcohol use: a systematic review of longitudinal studies. *Alcohol and Alcoholism*, 44(3):229–243.

Babor TF et al. (2010). *Alcohol: no ordinary commodity. Research and public policy,* 2nd ed. Oxford, Oxford University Press.

Booth A et al. (2008). *Independent review of the effects of alcohol pricing and promotion, Part A: Systematic Reviews*. London, Department of Health.

Collins RL, Ellickson PL, McCaffrey D (2007). Early adolescent exposure to alcohol advertising and its relationship to underage drinking. *Journal of Adolescent Health,* 40(6):527–534.

DiFranza JR et al. (2006). Tobacco promotion and the initiation of tobacco use: assessing the evidence for causality. *Pediatrics,* 117(6):e1237.

Ellickson PL et al. (2005). Does alcohol advertising promote adolescent drinking? Results from a longitudinal assessment. *Addiction,* 100(2):235–246.

Engels R et al. (2009). Alcohol portrayal on television affects actual drinking behaviour. *Alcohol and Alcoholism,* 44(3):244–249.

Fisher LB et al. (2007). Predictors of initiation of alcohol use among US adolescents: findings from a prospective cohort study. *Archives of Pediatrics and Adolescent Medicine,* 161(10):959–966.

Gallet CA (2007). The demand for alcohol: a meta-analysis of elasticities. *Australian Journal of Agricultural and Resource Economics,* 51(2):121–135.

Gordon R, Hastings G, Moodie C (2010). Alcohol marketing and young people's drinking: what the evidence base suggests for policy. *Journal of Public Affairs*, 10(1–2):88–101.

Gordon R, MacKintosh AM, Moodie C (2011). The impact of alcohol marketing on youth drinking behaviour: a two-stage cohort study. *Alcohol and Alcoholism,* 45(5):470–480.

Hanewinkel R, Sargent J (2009). Longitudinal study of exposure to entertainment media and alcohol use among German adolescents. *Pediatrics,* 123(3):989.

Harris JL et al. (2009). A crisis in the marketplace: how food marketing contributes to childhood obesity and what can be done. *Annual Review of Public Health,* 30:211–225.

Hastings G et al. (2003). *Review of research on the effects of food promotion to children*. Glasgow, University of Strathclyde.

Hastings G et al. (2010). Alcohol advertising: the last chance saloon: failure of self regulation of UK alcohol advertising. *British Medical Journal*, 340:184–186.

Henriksen L et al. (2008). Receptivity to alcohol marketing predicts initiation of alcohol use. *Journal of Adolescent Health,* 42(1):28–35.

Hurtz SQ et al. (2007). The relationship between exposure to alcohol advertising in stores, owning alcohol promotional items, and adolescent alcohol use. *Alcohol and Alcoholism,* 42(2):143–149.

Koordeman R, Anschutz DJ, Engels RCME (2009). Exposure to alcohol commercials in movie theaters affects actual alcohol consumption in young adult high weekly drinkers: an experimental study. *The American Journal on Addictions,* 20(3):285–291.

Koordeman R et al. (2011a). Effects of alcohol portrayals in movies on actual alcohol consumption: an observational experimental study. *Addiction,* 106(3):547–554.

Koordeman R et al. (2011b). Do we act upon what we see? Direct effects of alcohol cues in movies on young adults' alcohol drinking. *Alcohol and Alcoholism,* 46(4):393.

Lovato C et al. (2003). Impact of tobacco advertising and promotion on increasing adolescent smoking behaviours. *Cochrane Database of Systematic Reviews*, (4)CD003439.

McClure AC et al. (2006). Ownership of alcohol-branded merchandise and initiation of teen drinking. *American Journal of Preventive Medicine*, 30(4):277–283.

McClure AC et al. (2009). Alcohol-branded merchandise and its association with drinking attitudes and outcomes in US adolescents. *Archives of Pediatrics and Adolescent Medicine*, 163(3):211–217.

Morgenstern M et al. (2011). Attitudes as mediators of the longitudinal association between alcohol advertising and youth drinking. *Archives of Pediatrics and Adolescent Medicine*, 165(7):610.

Nelson JP (2003). Advertising bans, monopoly and alcohol demand: testing for substitution effects using state panel data. *Review of Industrial Organization*, 22:1–25.

Nelson JP (2010). Alcohol advertising bans, consumption, and control policies in seventeen OECD countries, 1975–2000. *Applied Economics*, 42:803–823.

Nestle M (2006). Food marketing and childhood obesity a matter of policy. *New England Journal of Medicine*, 354(24):2527–2529.

O'Brien KS et al. (2011). Alcohol industry and non-alcohol industry sponsorship of sportspeople and drinking. *Alcohol and Alcoholism*, 46(2):210.

Pasch KE et al. (2007). Outdoor alcohol advertising near schools: what does it advertise and how is it related to intentions and use of alcohol among young adolescents? *Journal of Studies on Alcohol and Drugs*, 68(4):587–596.

Paynter J, Edwards R (2009). The impact of tobacco promotion at the point of sale: a systematic review. *Nicotine & Tobacco Research*, 11(1):25–35.

Saffer H (1991). Alcohol advertising bans and alcohol abuse: an international perspective. *Journal of Health Economics*, 10(1):65–79.

Saffer H, Dave D (2004). Alcohol consumption and alcohol advertising bans. *Applied Economics*, 34:11.

Saffer H, Dave D (2006). *Alcohol advertising and alcohol consumption by adolescents. Health Economics*, 15(6):617–637.

Sargent J et al. (2006). Alcohol use in motion pictures and its relation with early-onset teen drinking. *Journal of Studies on Alcohol and Drugs*, 67(1):54–65.

Science Group of the European Alcohol and Health Forum (2009). *Does marketing communication impact on the volume and patterns of consumption of alcoholic beverages, especially by young people? –a review of longitudinal studies*. Brussels, European Commission, Directorate-General for Health and Consumers (http://ec.europa.eu/health/ph_determinants/life_style/alcohol/Forum/docs/science_o01_en.pdf, accessed 23 February 2012.

Smith LA, Foxcroft DR (2009). The effect of alcohol advertising, marketing and portrayal on drinking behaviour in young people: systematic review of prospective cohort studies. *BMC Public Health*, 9:51.

Snyder LB et al. (2006). Effects of alcohol advertising exposure on drinking among youth. *Archives of Pediatrics and Adolescent Medicine*, 160(1):18–24.

Stacy AW et al. (2004). Exposure to televised alcohol ads and subsequent adolescent alcohol use. *American Journal of Health Behavior*, 28(6):498–509.

Wellman RJ et al. (2006). The extent to which tobacco marketing and tobacco use in films contribute to children's use of tobacco: a meta-analysis. *Archives of Pediatrics and Adolescent Medicine*, 160(12):1285.

WHO Regional Office for Europe (2009). *Evidence for the effectiveness and cost–effectiveness of interventions to reduce alcohol-related harm*. Copenhagen, WHO Regional Office for Europe (http://www.euro.who.int/__data/assets/pdf_file/0020/43319/E92823.pdf, accessed 12 February 2012).

Pricing of alcohol

Esa Österberg

Introduction

The most common measure by which the public sector at local, state or national level has affected the economic availability of alcoholic beverages is taxation in its different forms. These include, among others, setting excise duties or value added taxes on alcoholic beverages. Historically, the most common reason for taxing alcoholic beverages has been to acquire financial resources for the public sector (Babor et al., 2010). However, the effects of price changes on alcohol consumption and related harm are the same regardless as to whether the changes in taxes – leading to price changes – are motivated by fiscal, social order or public health interests.

Besides taxing alcoholic beverages, there are other measures affecting the economic availability of alcohol such as minimum prices for alcoholic beverages or regulation of discount prices. Until recently, however, the primary research and policy attention has been directed towards tax levels, and the effects of tax and price changes are often not clearly distinguished.

The impact of changes in prices of alcoholic beverages on alcohol consumption and related harm has been more extensively studied than any other potential alcohol policy measure (Anderson & Baumberg, 2006). When other factors remain unchanged, an increase in alcohol prices generally leads to a decrease in alcohol consumption, and a decrease in alcohol prices usually leads to an increase in alcohol consumption (Anderson & Baumberg, 2006). As a rule, the effect of a change in prices of a certain magnitude has different effects on the consumption of different kinds of alcohol, for example, distilled spirits, wines and beer. Usually elasticity values also vary between countries, and their values may change within a country as time passes (see, for example, Bruun et al., 1975; Ornstein & Levy, 1983; Leung & Phelps, 1991; Edwards et al., 1994; Österberg, 1995; 2001; Leppänen, Sullström & Suoniemi, 2001). The addictive nature of alcohol implies that the short-term price elasticity of alcoholic beverages is smaller in absolute value than the long-term price elasticity (Anderson & Baumberg, 2006; Box 5).

Box 5. Price elasticity of alcoholic beverages

In econometric studies, the term "price elasticity" is used to express the effect of price changes on alcohol consumption. Negative own price elasticity value means that changes in prices and consumption are in the opposite direction: a rise in price leads to a decrease in consumption and a reduction in price leads to an increase in consumption. The numerical value of price elasticity gives the strength of the effect of a price change on consumption.

Alcoholic beverages are said to be price-elastic if the elasticity has an absolute value greater than one, which means that the percentage change in the amount of alcohol consumed is greater than the percentage change in price. If the price elasticity has a value of -1.5, it means that a 1% rise in alcohol price will reduce alcohol consumption by 1.5%.

If the elasticity has an absolute value smaller than one, alcoholic beverages are said to be price-inelastic. This means that the percentage change in the amount of alcohol consumed is smaller than the percentage change in price. If the price elasticity has a value of -0.5, it means that a 1% rise in alcohol price will decrease alcohol consumption by 0.5%.

Price inelasticity does not mean that consumption is not responsive to price changes. Rather, it means that the proportional change in consumption is smaller than the proportional change in price. Only if the price elasticity value is 0.0 will price changes have no effect on consumption.

A wide range of studies have shown that increasing the price of alcohol reduces both acute and chronic harm related to drinking among people of all ages. This kind of evidence indicates that heavy or problem drinkers are no exception to the basic rule that alcohol consumers respond to changes in alcohol prices (Babor et al., 2010).

Studies have found that increases in prices of alcoholic beverages disproportionately reduce alcohol consumption by young people, and also have a greater impact (in terms of alcohol intake) on more frequent and heavier drinkers than on less frequent and lighter drinkers (Anderson & Baumberg, 2006). Changes in alcohol prices have also been found to influence drinking to the point of intoxication.

Summary of recent evidence

Since 2006, three meta-analyses of the effects of changes in alcohol prices and taxes on drinking have been published (Table 11). The latest one, published in 2009 by Wagenaar and colleagues, is based on 112 studies reported in English (Wagenaar, Salois & Komro, 2009). The meta-analysis by Fogarty (2006) is based on elasticity estimates from those studies dealt with in Alcohol Policy and the Public Good, published in 1994 (Edwards et al., 1994; Fogarty, 2006). The analysis by Gallet (2007) includes 132 studies of alcohol price, income or advertising elasticities from 24 countries.

Table 11. Own-price elasticities for alcoholic beverages in three recent meta-analyses

Source	Distilled spirits	Wine	Beer	All alcoholic beverages
Fogarty, 2006	-0.70	-0.77	-0.38	N/A
Gallet, 2007	-0.68	-0.70	-0.36	-0.50
Wagenaar, Salois & Komro, 2009b	-0.80	-0.69	-0.46	-0.51

The explanation for the low absolute value of own-price elasticity for beer could be that beer is a common beverage consumed during everyday leisure activities or with meals in countries where the studies in these meta-analyses originate. In these countries beer may be viewed as a necessary commodity among beer drinkers. In some other countries, beer is more of a luxury item with higher price elasticity (Edwards et al., 1994). This point is highlighted in the case of wine, which seems overall to have a higher absolute value for own-price elasticity than beer. In countries where it is an ordinary beverage with meals, wine can, however, be quite price-inelastic, with a low absolute value (Edwards et al., 1994). On the other hand, not so many decades ago, wine was quite a rare luxury item in the Nordic countries, where it was used mostly on festive occasions. It is, therefore, no surprise that at that time wine had an own-price elasticity of -1.6 in Sweden, and in later years the price elasticity of wine has been -1.5 in Norway and -1.3 in Finland (Sundström & Ekström, 1962; Horverak, 1979; Salo, 1990).

As Wagenaar and colleagues emphasize, price elasticities are not inherent properties of alcoholic beverages (Wagenaar, Salois & Komro, 2009). In the same manner as different uses of alcoholic beverages are reflected in price elasticity values, so the substitution between different alcoholic beverages as well as other commodities mainly depends on the uses of alcoholic beverages (Bruun et al., 1975). For instance, in a country where wine is used as a beverage with meals, a substantial increase in wine prices could increase the consumption of bottled water but it would hardly increase the use of home-distilled spirits or illicit drugs. In countries where alcoholic beverages are mainly used as intoxicants, increases in alcohol prices are more likely to lead to an increase in the consumption of home-distilled or -brewed beverages or even illicit drugs than of bottled water or milk.

Besides the price elasticity for all alcoholic beverages of -0.50 in the short term, Gallet also found a long-term elasticity of -0.82 (Gallet, 2007). Furthermore, he examined the importance of income elasticities for the demand of alcoholic beverages. In his meta-analysis income elasticity for all alcoholic beverages is 0.50, meaning that a 1% increase in consumers' incomes leads to a 0.5% increase in alcohol consumption (Gallet, 2007).

One of the results in the meta-analysis by Wagenaar and colleagues is that price changes affect all types of beverage and all kinds of drinker, from light to heavy drinkers. According to their analyses, price and tax changes affect heavy drinking significantly, but the magnitude of the effect on heavy drinkers was less than on overall drinking (Wagenaar, Salois & Komro, 2009). In Switzerland, over four waves of panel data, Gmel and colleagues found that heavier drinkers increased their consumption more sharply in the short term but declined to the level before the tax change in the long term (Gmel et al., 2008). Furthermore, recent studies of the effects of tax changes on problem indicators provide strong evidence that changes in alcohol taxes do influence the rates of problem drinking (Babor et al., 2010). For instance, the reduction in alcohol taxation in Finland in 2004 had substantial effects on alcohol-related sudden deaths, overall alcohol-related mortality, and criminality and hospitalizations (Koski et al., 2007; Herttua, 2010; Mäkelä & Österberg, 2009). In Alaska, United States, excise duty increases in 1983 and 2002 were associated with substantial reductions in alcohol-related disease mortality (Wagenaar, Maldonado-Molina & Wagenaar, 2009).

Affordability

The term "alcohol affordability" is nowadays also frequently used. This refers to people's ability to buy and consume alcohol, and it is a function of alcohol price and consumers' income (Rabinovich et al., 2009). According to Rabinovich and colleagues, affordability of alcohol increased between 1996 and 2004 in almost all EU member states. Their analysis also indicated that across the EU, 84% of the increase in alcohol affordability in the period 1966–2004 was driven by increases in income, and only 16% was driven by changes in alcohol prices (Rabinovich et al., 2009). This is because while incomes have increased considerably across the EU countries, the relative prices of alcoholic beverages have remained relatively stable or fallen (Rabinovich et al., 2009).

In the period 1995–2010, developments in excise duty rates were not at all uniform. In some countries (mainly the Nordics), alcohol excise duty rates were lower in nominal terms in 2010 than in 1995. In some countries, Germany being the most important example, alcohol excise duty rates were held constant in nominal terms in the 1955–2010. In most of the countries belonging to the EU before May 2004, the nominal values of alcohol excise duty rates were increased but by less than the rate of inflation, meaning than even in these countries the real values of excise duties fell. Only in a few countries, such as Greece and Italy, the nominal values of excise duty rates were increased so much that the excise duty rates also increased in real terms (Österberg, 2011).

Countries that joined the EU in 2004, and later countries such as Bulgaria and Romania, had to increase their alcohol excise duty rates considerably before or when they joined the EU. In almost all new EU member states since 2003, the nominal and real values of alcohol excise duty rates increased between 2004 and 2010. The exceptions are Cyprus, with a constant nominal rate, and Malta, with a constant excise duty rate for beer and a 50% decrease for distilled spirits. Despite increases in alcohol excise duty rates in the new EU member states, the lowest excise duty rates were still found among them in 2011, Bulgaria and Romania being the clearest examples. Low excise duty rates for beer can also be found among the older member states (Germany, Luxembourg and Spain) (Österberg, 2011).

By 2011, no EU member states had moved from a zero excise duty rate for wine to a positive excise duty rate. In fact, during the creation of the single market in 1993 or in the process of joining it later, four countries (Bulgaria, Hungary, Luxembourg and Romania) abandoned their former positive duty rate for wine.

Minimum prices

A complementary measure to tax increases, and one which manages any lack of pass-through of tax to price, is to set a minimum price per gram of alcohol, a policy option with an impact on heavy consumers far in excess of that on light consumers. The impact has been tested in Canada (Stockwell et al., 2012), and modelled in the United Kingdom in England (Purshouse et al., 2009) and Scotland (ScHARR, 2010), where there is currently a law before the Scottish Parliament to introduce a minimum price for alcohol of €0.07/g alcohol (Scottish Government, 2012).

Minimum alcohol prices in British Columbia, Canada, were adjusted intermittently over the years 1989–2010. Time-series and longitudinal models of aggregate alcohol consumption with price and other economic data as independent variables found that a 10% increase in the minimum price of an alcoholic beverage reduced its consumption relative to other beverages by 16.1% (Stockwell et al., 2012). Time-series estimates indicated that a 10% increase in minimum prices reduced the consumption of spirits and liqueurs by 6.8%, wine by 8.9%, alcoholic sodas and ciders by 13.9%, beer by 1.5% and all alcoholic drinks by 3.4%.

In England, 59% of the alcohol sold for consumption elsewhere ("off trade") and 14% of the alcohol sold for consumption on the premises ("on trade") is sold for less than 5 pence (£0.05/€0.06) per gram of alcohol (Purshouse et al., 2009). Modelling estimated that setting a minimum price of 5 p/g (€0.06/g) would reduce overall consumption by 2.6% (a 3.4 g reduction per week), affecting heavy drinkers far more (25 g/week) than moderate drinkers (0.01 g/week). It was estimated that annual deaths would decline by 157 in the first year and by 1381 after 10 years. Annual hospital admissions would fall by an estimated 6300 in the first year and by 40 800 after 10 years. The intervention would also lead to an estimated decline of 16 000 criminal offences during the 10 years modelled. During the same period, the study predicted that there would be 12 400 fewer unemployed people and 100 000 fewer sick days. The study estimated the value of these reductions in harm to society as £5.4 billion (€6.2 billion) over 10 years. The estimated value of this minimum price policy for the first year included National Health Service savings (£25 million/€29 million), the value of quality-adjusted life-years (QALYs) gained through better health (£63 million/€72 million), savings related to the costs of crime (£17 million/€19 million), the value of crime QALYs gained (£21 million/€24 million) and employment-related benefits (£312 million/€356 million). Again, the cost impact of this policy on consumers varied substantially among different groups of drinkers. It would cost drinkers an estimated £22 (€25) per year, ranging from £106 (€121) for heavy drinkers down to £6 (€7) for moderate drinkers. If no changes were made to consumption, it would cost heavy drinkers an estimated additional £138 (€157) per annum and moderate drinkers an estimated additional £6 (€7).

Symmetry of price elasticities

It has been argued that, because of the addictive nature of alcohol, price elasticities of alcoholic beverages may not be symmetrical (Bruun et al., 1975). In other words, a decrease of a certain magnitude in alcohol prices may have a greater impact on alcohol consumption than the same magnitude of price increase realized afterwards (see Box 6). Another reason for asymmetrical price elasticities could be that alcoholic beverages are so easily available that a further increase in alcohol availability will not increase alcohol consumption because the market is already saturated. Saturation has also been used as one explanation for the results in the Nordic alcohol tax study (Room et al., 2012).

Box 6. Alcohol tax changes in Finland in 2004–2010

In March 2004, Finland reduced its alcohol excise duty rates by an average of 33%. The motivation for this decrease was that in May 2004, Estonia, which had much lower alcohol prices than Finland, joined the EU. As quantitative quotas for travellers' tax-free alcohol imports for own use from other EU member states had been abolished in January 2004, it was feared that private alcohol imports from Estonia would greatly reduce the amount of state-collected alcohol taxes as well as alcohol-related employment in Finland.

In 2005, total alcohol consumption per capita was 12% higher than in 2003. Despite the tax decreases, alcohol imports by travellers doubled between 2003 and 2005 and their share of total alcohol consumption rose to 17% in 2005. Meanwhile, domestic sales of alcoholic beverages increased. Despite a 7% increase in domestic alcohol sales from 2003 to 2005, the state collected 29% less excise duty on alcoholic beverages in 2005 than in 2003.

In 2008 and 2009, alcohol excise duty rates were increased three times, by an average of about 10% each time. Between 2007 and 2010, total alcohol consumption fell by 3% and alcohol imports by travellers rose by 11%. Despite the 7% decrease in domestic sales of alcoholic beverages between 2007 and 2010, the state collected 27% more alcohol excise duties in 2010 than in 2007.

These data show that consumption went up by 12% when taxes fell by 33% on average, but went down by only 3% when taxes went up about 30%, an example of asymmetry in elasticities.

The Nordic alcohol tax study dealt with Denmark, Finland and Sweden, which were all forced to abolish their quantitative quotas for travellers' alcohol imports from other EU member states at the beginning of 2004 (Karlsson & Österberg, 2009). In order to combat increases in alcohol imports by travellers, alcohol excise duty rates for distilled spirits were reduced in Denmark in October 2003. In Finland, excise duty rates were decreased for all alcoholic beverages in March 2004 (Box 6). In Denmark, neither the alcohol sales statistics nor the survey data found an increase in total alcohol consumption and there were no clear increases in mortality or morbidity series. The picture was much the same for the effects in Southern Sweden where an increase in travellers' alcohol imports from Denmark was expected (Room et al., 2012). Only in Finland was there found evidence of increases in alcohol consumption and related harm (Box 6).

Conclusions for policy and practice

Recent research evidence with regard to the economic availability of alcohol confirms previous knowledge and does not alter the fundamental conclusions of Bruun and colleagues in 1975. As Wagenaar and colleagues conclude their meta-analysis: "Results confirm previous reviews of this literature, but extend results in important ways ... Price affects drinking in all types of beverages and across the population of drinkers from light drinkers to heavy drinkers" (Wagenaar, Salois & Komro, 2009b).

The effects of prices as measured with price elasticities differ both across countries and different time periods as well as with regard to different categories of alcoholic beverage. These differences are related to the use values of alcoholic beverages and consumers' preferences as well as the actual uses of such beverages. Local drinking habits should, therefore, be taken into account when alcohol policy measures that affect the economic availability of alcohol are planned.

References

Anderson P, Baumberg B (2006). *Alcohol in Europe. A public health perspective*. London, Institute of Alcohol Studies.

Babor TF et al. (2010). *Alcohol: no ordinary commodity. Research and public policy,* 2nd ed. Oxford, Oxford University Press.

Bruun K et al. (1975). *Alcohol control policies in public health perspective*. Helsinki, Finnish Foundation for Alcohol Studies.

Edwards G et al. (1994). *Alcohol policy and the public good.* Oxford, Oxford University Press.

Fogarty J (2006). The nature of the demand for alcohol: understanding elasticity. *British Food Journal*, 108:316–332.

Gallet CA (2007). The demand for alcohol: a meta-analysis of elasticities. *The Australian Journal of Agricultural and Resource Economics*, 51:121–135.

Gmel G et al. (2008). Estimating regression to the mean and true effects of an intervention in a four-wave panel study. *Addiction,* 103:32–41.

Herttua K (2010). *The effects of the 2004 reduction in the price of alcohol and alcohol-related harm in Finland. A natural experiment based on register data*. Helsinki, The Family Federation of Finland.

Horverak Ø (1979). *Norsk alkoholpolitik 1960–1975 [Norwegian alcohol policy 1960–1975].* Oslo, Statens Institutt for Alkoholforskning.

Karlsson T, Österberg E (2009). *Alcohol affordability and cross-border trade in alcohol.* Östersund, Swedish National Institute of Public Health.

Koski A et al. (2007). Alcohol tax cuts and increase in alcohol-positive sudden deaths – a time-series intervention analysis. *Addiction,* 102:362–368.

Leppänen K, Sullström R, Suoniemi I (2001). *The consumption of alcohol in fourteen European countries. A comparative econometric analysis*. Helsinki, Stakes.

Leung S, Phelps C (1991). My kingdom for drink. A review of estimates of the price sensitivity of demand for alcoholic beverages. In: Hilton ME, Bloss G, eds. *Economics and the prevention of alcohol-related problems*. Rockville, MD, US Department of Health and Human Services, National Institute on Alcohol Abuse and Alcoholism:1–32.

Mäkelä P, Österberg E (2009). Weakening of one more alcohol control pillar: a review of the effects of the alcohol tax cuts in Finland in 2004. *Addiction,* 104:554–563.

Ornstein SI, Levy D (1983). Price and income elasticities and the demand for alcoholic beverages. In: Galanter M. *Recent developments in alcoholism*. New York, Plenum:303–345.

Österberg E (1995). Do alcohol prices affect consumption and related problems? In: Holder HD, Edwards G, eds. *Alcohol and public policy: evidence and issues*. Oxford, Oxford University Press:145–163.

Österberg E (2001). Effects of price and taxation. In: Heather N, Peters TJ, Stockwell T, eds. *International handbook of alcohol dependence and problems*. Chichester, John Wiley and Sons, Ltd.: 685–698.

Österberg E (2011). Alcohol tax changes and the use of alcohol in Europe. *Drug and Alcohol Review*, 30:124–129.

Purshouse R et al. (2009). *Modelling to assess the effectiveness and cost–effectiveness of public health related strategies and interventions to reduce alcohol attributable harm in England using the Sheffield Alcohol Policy Model version 2.0. Report to the NICE Public Health Programme Development Group*. Sheffield, University of Sheffield, School of Health and Related Research (ScHARR).

Rabinovich L et al. (2009). *The affordability of alcoholic beverages in the European Union. Understanding the link between alcohol affordability, consumption and harms*. Cambridge, RAND Europe.

Room R et al. (2002). *Alcohol in developing societies: a public health approach*. Helsinki, Finnish Foundation for Alcohol Studies.

Salo M (1990). *Alkoholijuomien vähittäiskulutuksen analyysi vuosilta 1969–1988 [An analysis of off-premise retail sales of alcoholic beverages, 1969–1988]*. Helsinki, Alko.

Scottish Government (2012). Alcohol – minimum pricing [web site]. Edinburgh, The Scottish Government (http://www.scotland.gov.uk/Topics/Health/health/Alcohol/minimum-pricing, accessed 23 February 2012).

ScHARR (2010). *Model-based appraisal of alcohol minimum pricing and off-licensed trade discount bans in Scotland using the Sheffield Alcohol Policy Model (v2): an update based on newly available data*. Sheffield, University of Sheffield, School of Health and Related Research (ScHARR) (http://www.scotland.gov.uk/Publications/2010/04/20091852/0, accessed 23 February 2012).

Stockwell T et al. (2012). Does minimum pricing reduce alcohol consumption? The experience of a Canadian province *Addiction*, doi: 10.1111/j.1360-0443.2011.03763.x

Sundström Å, Ekström J (1962). *Dryckeskonsumtionen i Sverige [Beverage consumption in Sweden]*. Stockholm, Industrins Utredningsinstitut.

Wagenaar AC, Maldonado-Molina MM, Wagenaar BH (2009). Effects of alcohol tax increases on alcohol-related disease mortality in Alaska: time-series analyses from 1976 to 2004. *American Journal of Public Health*, 99:1464–1470.

Wagenaar AC, Salois MJ, Komro KA (2009). Effects of beverage alcohol price and tax levels on drinking: a meta-analysis of 1003 estimates from 112 studies. *Addiction*, 104:179–190.

Overview of effectiveness and cost–effectiveness

Peter Anderson and Lars Møller

Introduction[7]

The report *Alcohol in Europe. A public health perspective*, prepared in 2006 for the EC (Anderson & Baumberg, 2006), grouped alcohol policies under five headings: (i) policies that reduce drinking and driving; (ii) policies that support education, communication, training and public awareness; (iii) policies that regulate the alcohol market; (iv) policies that support the reduction of harm in drinking and surrounding environments; and (v) policies that support interventions for individuals. Based on the then available evidence, it concluded the following.

- The drink–driving policies that are highly effective include unrestricted (random) breath-testing, lowered BAC levels, administrative licence suspension and lower BAC levels for young drivers. The limited evidence did not find an impact from designated driver and safe drive programmes. Alcohol interlocks can be effective as a preventive measure, but as a measure with drink–driving offenders they only work as long as they are fitted to a vehicle. It was estimated that, compared with no testing, implementation of unrestricted breath-testing as a policy to prevent drink–driving would avert an estimated 111 000 years of disability and premature death throughout the EU at an estimated cost of €233 million each year.

- Policies that support education, communication, training and public awareness have a low impact. Although the reach of school-based educational programmes can be high because of the captive audiences in schools, the population impact of these programmes is small owing to their current limited or lack of effectiveness. Recommendations exist as to how the effectiveness of school-based programmes might be improved. On the other hand, mass media programmes have a particular role to play in reinforcing community awareness of the problems created by alcohol use and to prepare the ground for specific interventions.

- There is very strong evidence for the effectiveness of policies that regulate the alcohol market in reducing the harm done by alcohol, including taxation and managing the physical availability of alcohol (limiting times of sale and raising the minimum drinking age). Alcohol taxes are particularly important in targeting young people and the harm done by alcohol. The evidence shows that if opening hours for the sale of alcohol are extended, more violent harm results. Restricting the volume and content of commercial communication of alcohol products is likely to reduce harm. Advertisements have a particular impact in promoting a more positive attitude to drinking among young people. It was estimated that, compared with no tax on alcohol, the current level of tax with a 25% increase in the tax rate throughout the EU would avert an estimated 656 000 years of disability and premature death at an estimated cost of €159 million each year; reducing the availability of alcohol from retail outlets by a 24-hour period each week would avert an estimated 123 000 years of disability and premature death at an estimated implementation cost of €98 million each year; and banning the advertising of alcohol would avert an estimated 202 000 years of disability and premature death at an estimated implementation cost of €95 million each year.

- There is growing evidence for the impact of strategies that alter the drinking context in reducing the harm done by alcohol. These strategies are, however, primarily applicable to drinking in bars and restaurants, and their effectiveness relies on adequate enforcement. They are also more effective when backed up by community-based prevention programmes.

---

[7] In this chapter, unless stated otherwise, Europe refers to the countries covered by the WHO European Region.

- There is extensive evidence for the impact of brief advice, particularly in primary care settings, in reducing harmful alcohol consumption. Providing such primary care-based brief advice to 25% of the at-risk population would avert an estimated 408 000 years of disability and premature death at an estimated cost of €740 million each year.

- Implementing a comprehensive EU-wide package of effective policies and programmes that included random breath-testing, taxation, restricted access, an advertising ban and brief advice from a doctor, was estimated to cost European governments €1.3 billion to implement (about 1% of the total tangible costs of alcohol to society and only about 10% of the estimated income gained from a 10% rise in the price of alcohol due to taxes in the countries belonging to the EU before May 2004), and was estimated to avoid 1.4 million years of disability and premature death a year, equivalent to 2.3% of all disability and premature death facing the EU.

Summary of recent evidence

Since 2006, considerable evidence has been gained on the effectiveness and cost–effectiveness of alcohol policies. This evidence has been summarized in a range of publications (Anderson, Chisholm & Fuhr, 2009; Anderson et al., 2011; Babor et al., 2010; WHO Regional Office for Europe, 2009a; 2009b; 2010). As described in the previous chapters, what is clear about the change in evidence over time is that there are now many more publications of systematic reviews and meta-analyses which have strengthened the conclusions of previous reviews.

WHO's CHOosing Interventions that are Cost Effective (CHOICE) model provides estimates of the costs of implementing certain policies and estimates of the benefits likely to be accrued. Although based on the best available implementation costs at the country level and on the best available evidence for implementation effects, they are, of course, just models. However, they do give policy-oriented guidelines for the most likely cost–effective approaches for improving health. Full details and technical information can be found on the CHOICE website (WHO, 2012). A summary of the estimated implementation costs and impact of different alcohol policy interventions, compared to a Europe with none of these policies, is shown in Table 12, with an estimate of the cost per DALY saved summarized in Fig. 18 (WHO Regional Office for Europe, 2009a). It should be remembered in all economic analyses of alcohol policies that, although tax increases bring in extra revenue for governments, economists regard these revenues as revenue-neutral, since the money raised can be rebated to consumers by allowing an equal reduction in other taxes, such as income taxes.

For information and education, and community action, the costs of school-based education and mass-media awareness campaigns have been estimated respectively. Although these interventions are not expensive, they do not notably alter consumption levels or health outcomes.

In relation to the health sector response, the estimated cost–effectiveness of such interventions is not as favourable as the population-level policy instruments summarized below because they require direct contact with health care professionals and services. Although brief interventions are the most expensive to implement, it should be noted that within health service expenditure, brief interventions for hazardous and harmful alcohol consumption are one of the most cost–effective of all health service interventions in leading to improved health. Where drink–driving policies and countermeasures are concerned, the estimated cost–effectiveness ranged from I$ 781 (in Eur-C countries) to I$ 4625 (in Eur-B countries).

Table 12. Costs, impact and cost–effectiveness of different policy options in three subregions of the WHO European Region

Target area specific intervention(s)	Coverage (%)	Eur-A[a]			Eur-B[b]			Eur-C[c]		
		Annual cost per million persons (I$ million)[d]	Annual effect per million persons (DALYs saved)	I$ per DALY saved[e]	Annual cost per million persons (I$ million)[d]	Effect per million persons per year (DALYs saved)	I$ per DALY saved[e]	Annual cost per million persons (I$ millions)[d]	Effect per million persons per year (DALYs saved)	I$ per DALY saved[e]
ising and political										
education	80	0.84	—	N/A*	0.70	—	N/A*	0.34	—	N/A*
response										
ons for heavy drinkers	30	4.20	672	6256	0.77	365	2100	1.78	667	2671
ction										
ampaigns	80	0.83	—	N/A*	0.95	—	N/A*	0.79	—	N/A*
policies and ures										
egislation and enforcement eath-testing campaigns)	80	0.77	204	3762	0.74	160	4625	0.72	917	781
alcohol										
ss to retail outlets	80	0.78	316	2475	0.56	414	1360	0.47	828	567
lcoholic beverages										
e advertising ban	95	0.78	351	2226	0.56	224	2509	0.47	488	961
es										
se taxation by 20%	95	1.09	2301	472	0.92	726	1272	0.67	1759	380
se taxation by 50%	95	1.09	2692	404	0.92	852	1083	0.67	1995	335
nt, 20% less unrecorded	95	1.94	2069	939	1.26	706	1780	0.87	1741	498
nt, 50% less unrecorded	95	2.21	2137	1034	1.34	790	1692	0.93	1934	480

w adult mortality and very low child mortality): Andorra, Austria, Belgium, Croatia, Cyprus, Czech Republic, Denmark, Finland, France, Germany, Greece, Iceland Italy, Luxembourg, Malta, Monaco, Netherlands, Norway, Portugal, San Marino, Slovenia, Spain, Sweden, Switzerland, United Kingdom.
dult mortality and low child mortality): Albania, Armenia, Azerbaijan, Bosnia and Herzegovina, Bulgaria, Georgia, Kyrgyzstan, Montenegro, Poland, Romania, Serbia stan, The former Yugoslav Republic of Macedonia, Turkey, Turkmenistan, Uzbekistan.
dult mortality and low child mortality): Belarus, Estonia, Hungary, Kazakhstan, Latvia, Lithuania, Republic of Moldova, Russian Federation, Ukraine.
n cost in 2005 international dollars (I$).
ness ratio, expressed in terms of international dollars per DALY saved.

Fig. 18. Cost–effectiveness estimates, in I$/DALY gained, for various forms of alcohol policy action in three subregions of the WHO European Region

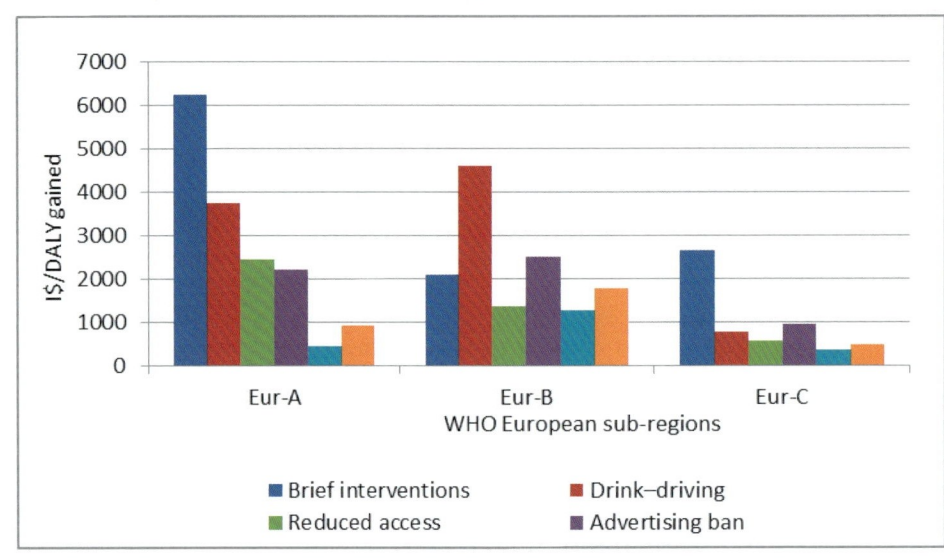

Note. Cost–effectiveness is inversely proportional to the height of the bars. For a description of each action used in the calculations, see Anderson, 2009b.

Reducing access to retail outlets for specified periods of the week and implementing a comprehensive advertising ban are estimated to have the potential to be cost–effective countermeasures, but only if they are fully enforced (each healthy year of life restored costs between I$ 567 and I$ 2509).

Tax increases (of 20% or even 50%) are estimated to be highly cost–effective throughout Europe. Even accounting for longer life, and thus potentially increased social welfare costs, taxation remains a highly cost–effective alcohol policy option. The effect of alcohol tax increases could be mitigated by illegal production, tax evasion and illegal trading, which account for approximately 12% of all consumption in Eur-A countries and 40% in Eur-B and Eur-C countries. Reducing this unrecorded consumption (by 20–50%) via concerted tax enforcement efforts is estimated to cost 50–100% more than a tax increase but to produce similar levels of effect. In settings with higher levels of unrecorded production and consumption, increasing the proportion of consumption that is taxed (and therefore more costly to the price-sensitive consumer) may represent a more effective pricing policy than a simple increase in excise tax, which may only encourage further illegal production, smuggling and cross-border purchases.

Figs. 19–21 plot the total costs and effects of each single and combined intervention on an expansion curve. The lower right boundary of this plot represents the increasing incremental cost of saving one additional DALY and indicates the most efficient way of combining different strategies. Interventions to the north-west of this cost–effectiveness frontier or expansion path are "dominated", i.e. they are less effective and/or more costly than (a combination of) other interventions. The most cost–effective options are those that occur on the inflections of the expansion path. In all three subregions of Europe, the most cost–effective option is increased taxation (current + 50%); followed by increased tax and scaled-up tax enforcement in Eur-A and Eur-C countries and increased tax and reduced access in Eur-B countries; followed by increased tax, scaled-up tax enforcement and reduced access in all three subregions; followed by increased tax, scaled-up tax enforcement, reduced access, an advertising ban and brief advice in all three subregions.

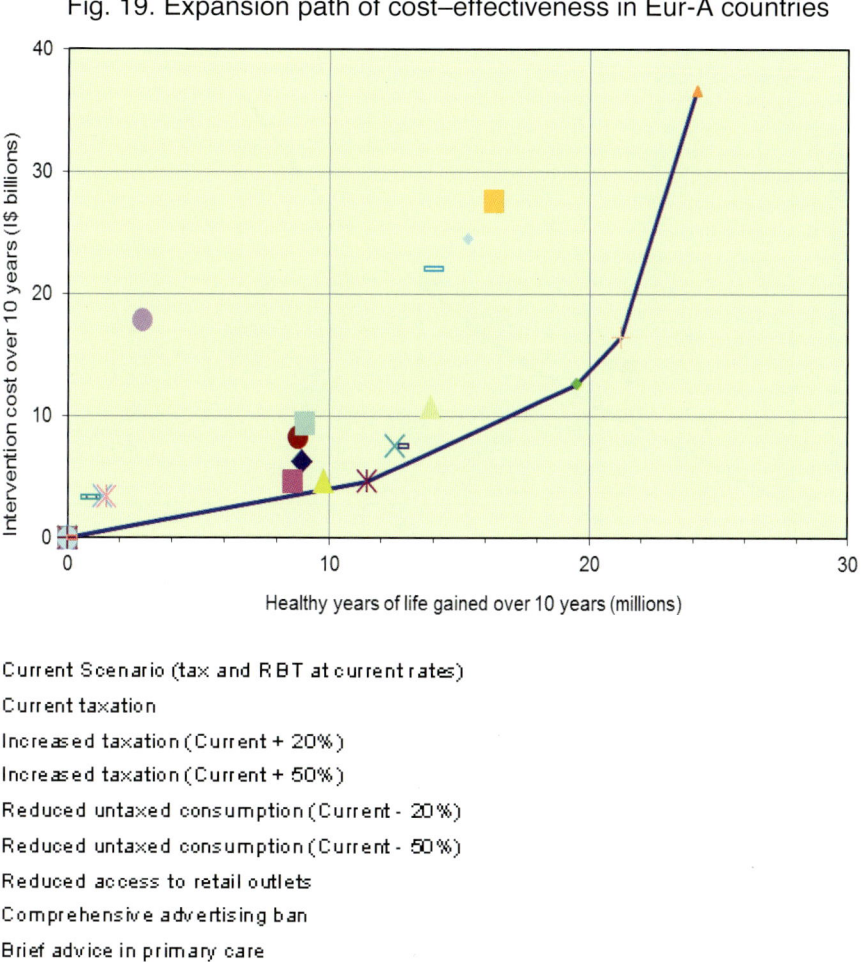

Fig. 19. Expansion path of cost–effectiveness in Eur-A countries

- Current Scenario (tax and RBT at current rates)
- Current taxation
- Increased taxation (Current + 20%)
- Increased taxation (Current + 50%)
- Reduced untaxed consumption (Current - 20%)
- Reduced untaxed consumption (Current - 50%)
- Reduced access to retail outlets
- Comprehensive advertising ban
- Brief advice in primary care
- Roadside breath-testing (fatal injuries only)
- Roadside breath-testing (including non-fatal injuries)
- Combination 1: Increased tax and scaled-up tax enforcement
- Combination 2: Increased tax and reduced access
- Combination 3: Increased tax and Advertising Ban
- Combination 4: Increased tax and Brief advice
- Combination 5: Increased tax + Ad Ban + Brief advice
- Combination 6: Increased tax + Ad Ban + Reduced access
- Combination 7: Increased tax + Reduced access + Tax enforcement
- Combination 8: Increased tax + Brief Advice + Ad ban + Reduced access
- Combination 9: Increased tax + Brief Advice + Ad ban + Reduced access + Tax enforcement

Importantly for policy discussions, it should be noted that the current intervention mix (■), does not appear on any of the expansion paths, indicating room for improvement from a cost–effectiveness point of view, and that more DALYs could, therefore, be saved by increasing the taxation level, and improving coverage of interventions and enforcement, possibly even in the current budgetary range using resource re-allocation.

Finally, it should be noted that a comprehensive policy that combines individual elements can be far more cost–effective than the individual policy elements alone. For example, current taxation plus a 50% increase, which lies at the first inflexion of the expansions path in Eur-A has an incremental and average cost–effectiveness of I$ 404/DALY averted. The next inflection (increased tax and scaled-up enforcement) has an incremental cost–effectiveness of I$ 991 and

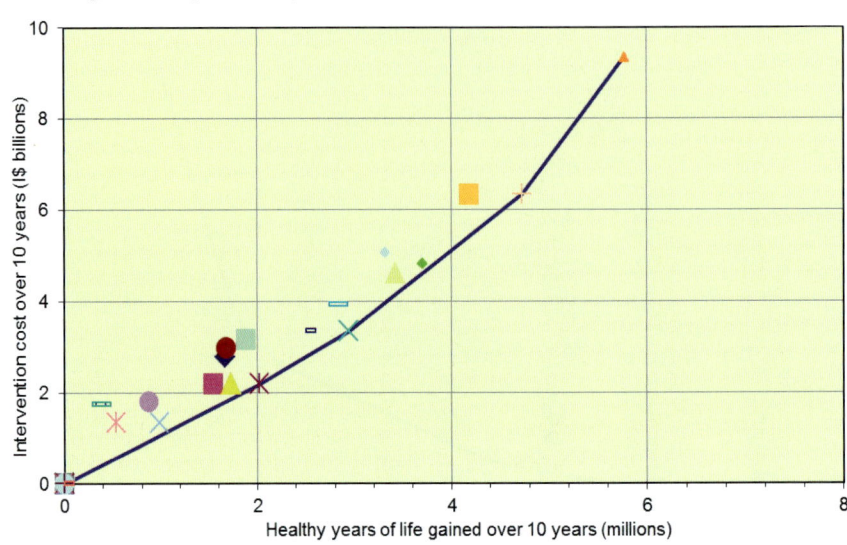

Fig. 20. Expansion path of cost–effectiveness in Eur-B countries

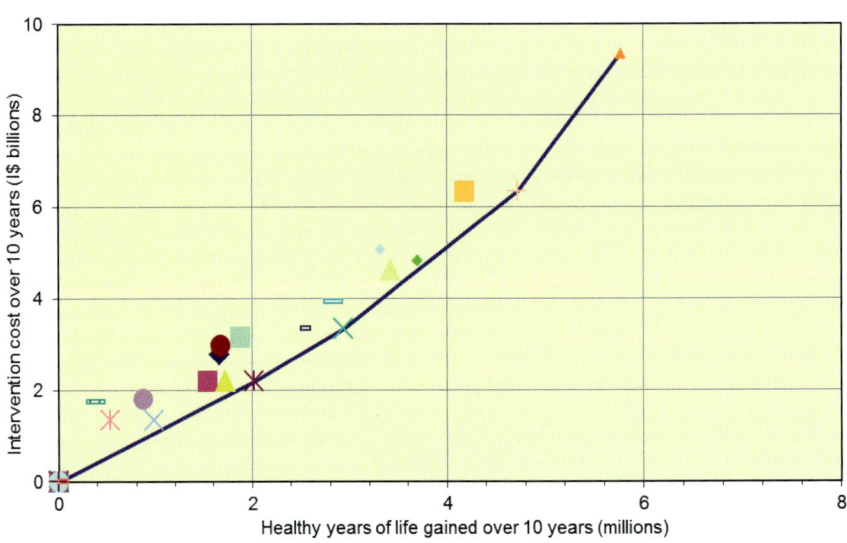

Fig. 21. Expansion path of cost–effectiveness in Eur-C countries

an average cost–effectiveness of I$ 647. The third inflection (increased tax, scaled-up enforcement and reduced access) has an incremental cost–effectiveness of I$ 2252 and an average cost–effectiveness of I$ 776. The final point (increased tax, scaled-up enforcement, reduced access, advertising ban and brief advice) has an incremental cost–effectiveness of I$ 6923 and an average cost–effectiveness of I$ 1517.

Avoidable-burden analyses

Recently initiatives have been started to undertake avoidable-burden studies, which estimate the existing health or economic burden due to alcohol that could be avoided through strengthened alcohol policy measures. In England, for example, research has been funded to extend a cost–effectiveness analysis to model the impact of specified policy changes on outcomes beyond just health (Purshouse et al., 2009). The model estimates suggest that a 10% increase in the price of alcoholic beverages would reduce alcohol consumption by 4.4%, an average reduction of 5.5 g alcohol per week, with a significantly greater reduction of 25 g per week for heavy drinkers (defined as men who drink more than 400 g alcohol per week and women who drink more than 280 g/week) than the 4 g/week reduction for moderate drinkers (men who drink up to 168 g alcohol per week and women who drink up to 112 g/week). The research estimated that in England (population 51 million), the annual number of deaths would fall by 232 within the first year and 1681 after 10 years. In addition, hospital admissions would decline by an estimated 10 100 in the initial year, reaching full effect after 10 years with 50 800 admissions avoided annually. The study also predicted that a 10% price increase would reduce the number of criminal offences by 65 000 over the course of a decade, with a savings in the direct costs of crime of £70 million (€80 million at the August 2009 exchange rate) per year. In the workplace, it was anticipated that the same intervention would mean 12 800 fewer unemployed people and 310 000 fewer sick days over 10 years. The estimated total value of this price increase is £7.8 billion (€8.9 billion) (when discounted[8]) over the 10 years modelled. The breakdown of the estimated value for the first year include National Health Service savings (£43 million, or €49 million), the value of quality-adjusted life years (QALYs)[9] gained through better health (£119 million/€136 million)), crime costs saved (£70 million/€80 million), the value of QALYs gained through crime reduction (£98 million/€112 million) and employment-related benefits (£330 million/€376 million). The direct cost to consumers would vary significantly among different types of drinker. The overall figure is £33 (€38) per drinker per annum, ranging from an estimated £116 (€132) annually for heavy drinkers to £17 (€19) for moderate drinkers.

The EU has funded a number of projects on cost–effectiveness (see Annex 4).

Conclusions for policy and practice

There is now a substantial evidence base of systematic reviews and meta-analyses which show that policies that regulate the environment in which alcohol is marketed (particularly its price and availability) are effective in reducing alcohol-related harm. Enforced legislative measures to reduce drinking and driving and interventions directed individually towards at-risk drinkers are also effective. On the other hand, school-based education is found not to reduce alcohol-related harm, although public information and educational programmes have a role in providing information and in increasing attention to and acceptance of alcohol on the political and public agendas. Making alcohol more expensive and less available are highly cost–effective strategies to reduce harm. Banning alcohol advertising, introducing drink–driving countermeasures and directing individual interventions to at-risk drinkers are also cost–effective. In countries with relatively high levels of unrecorded production and consumption, an increase in the proportion of alcohol that is taxed may be a more effective pricing policy than a simple increase in tax.

Given that the benefits substantially exceed the costs, any remaining concerns over the distribution of benefits and costs must be concerns about equity and fairness, rather than efficiency and effectiveness. Here, it should be noted that gram for gram of alcohol consumed, individuals who are socially disadvantaged, whether by income, education or social capital, experience more harm from alcohol than those who are less socially disadvantaged. A price decrease in Finland in the early 2000s led to a 10% increase in per capita consumption and an increase in overall alcohol-related mortality of 16% among men and 31% among women

---

[8] In the analysis, costs were discounted at 3.5% annually according to standard English Department of Health practice, which means that future values are worth less than current values.
[9] QALYs and DALYs are similar measures of disease burden.

(Herttua, Mäkelä & Martikainen, 2008). Among people aged 30–59 years, the increased overall alcohol-related mortality in absolute terms was greatest among the unemployed or early pensioners and those with low education, social class or income. Those in employment and those aged over 35 years did not suffer from increased alcohol-related mortality during the two years after the change. Thus, a reciprocal relationship might be expected, with greater decreases in alcohol-related mortality among the disadvantaged following an increase in tax.

Implementing alcohol policy in many EU countries is often a matter of recovering a lost policy tradition that was abandoned during the deregulatory phase of the past three or so decades. A coordinated approach to delivering comprehensive policy would also reveal how well the models presented in this and other chapters behave, and therefore how to improve them.

References

Anderson P, Baumberg B (2006). *Alcohol in Europe. A public health perspective*. London, Institute of Alcohol Studies.

Anderson P, Chisholm D, Fuhr DC (2009). Effectiveness and cost–effectiveness of policies and programmes to reduce the harm caused by alcohol. *Lancet,* 373:2234–2246.

Anderson P et al. (2011). Communicating alcohol narratives: Creating a healthier relation with alcohol. *Journal of Health Communication*, 16(S2):27–36.

Babor TF et al. (2010). *Alcohol: no ordinary commodity. Research and public policy,* 2nd ed. Oxford, Oxford University Press.

Herttua K, Mäkelä P, Martikainen P (2008). Changes in alcohol-related mortality and its socioeconomic differences after a large reduction in prices: a natural experiment based on register data. *American Journal of Epidemiology*, 168(10):1110–1118.

Purshouse R et al. (2009). *Modelling to assess the effectiveness and cost–effectiveness of public health related strategies and interventions to reduce alcohol attributable harm in England using the Sheffield Alcohol Policy Model version 2.0. Report to the NICE Public Health Programme Development Group.* Sheffield, University of Sheffield, School of Health and Related Research (ScHARR).

WHO (2012). WHO-CHOICE [web site]. Geneva, World Health Organization (http://www.who.int/choice/en/, accessed 23 February 2012).

WHO Regional Office for Europe (2009a). *Evidence for the effectiveness and cost–effectiveness of interventions to reduce alcohol-related harm*. Copenhagen, WHO Regional Office for Europe.

WHO Regional Office for Europe (2009b). *Handbook for action to reduce alcohol-related harm*. Copenhagen, WHO Regional Office for Europe.

WHO Regional Office for Europe (2010). *European status report on alcohol and health 2010*. Copenhagen, WHO Regional Office for Europe (http://www.euro.who.int/__data/assets/pdf_file/0004/128065/e94533.pdf, accessed 14 February 2012).

Common evidence base and monitoring

Jacek Moskalewicz

Introduction

Existing evidence shows that having a national alcohol policy by itself has a low impact on the alcohol burden. According to Karlsson & Österberg (2007), who analysed the impact of seven policy measures on alcohol consumption, only 2.5% of the overall impact can be attributed to the existence of national programmes or action plans compared to a 40% contribution from tax policies or 30% from restrictions on alcohol sales. One likely factor is that national programmes do not recommend evidence-based measures that may affect state or private economic interests (Gordon & Anderson, 2011).

Monitoring and evaluation of the implementation and effectiveness of alcohol policy programmes and action plans seem to be crucial to strengthen their impact (WHO Regional Office for Europe, 2011a). However, implementation and evaluation reports (if they exist at all) rarely feed into the development of consecutive plans or programmes. Usually a new programme, like its precedents, is the result of a compromise between economic and health interests.

Monitoring approaches and their limitations

Statistics

Statistics for health, economic and other harm seem to be the most reliable as they have usually been in use for decades, are provided by well-established government agencies and are relatively well standardized, thanks to numerous international agencies. In addition, some agencies, including the EC and WHO, retrieve, clean and additionally standardize collected statistics. No matter their technical accuracy, however, statistical sources are human products and as such are heavily culture-specific or biased.

Sales statistics, which usually serve as the source for estimation of recorded consumption, often suffer from underestimation of real consumption owing to the existence of other sources of supply. These may be licit (such as duty-free quotas allowed for individual consumption, home production allowed to certain limits in many European countries or non-beverage alcohol bought for individual consumption) or illicit (including smuggling, illegal production, conversion of contaminated ethanol to drinkable fluid for sale as a regular drink, as well as reimported and untaxed alcohol from the legal alcohol industry). In the EU plus Norway, Switzerland and the EU candidate countries, the unrecorded share can vary from a few per cent to more than 35% of overall consumption (Annex 1).

Morbidity statistics can be affected by the level of development of alcohol treatment, as the more specialized the treatment, the greater the chance of being diagnosed as suffering from an alcohol-related disorder. On the other hand, in most countries, alcohol-related diagnoses are stigmatizing. Physicians may, therefore, be reluctant to put causes such as alcoholic liver cirrhosis or acute withdrawal on a death certificate. Time series can be, and in fact are, heavily affected by subsequent changes in the International Classification of Diseases (ICD); for example, the transition from ICD 9 to ICD 10 in Poland was followed by a significant drop in first hospital admissions due to alcoholic psychoses as physicians found a new convenient symbol (F10) without any specification for those who had previously been diagnosed as psychotics.

Surveys

Surveys, in particular broad data collection efforts by international agencies, may also be affected by the varying competence of the government officials who are supposed to respond. Sometimes information may not be reported in order to hide failures in alcohol policy, or some achievements over-emphasized so as to stress the success of a given policy or certain individuals or the reporting agency.

Neither do population surveys constitute an entirely reliable monitoring tool. The major issue is the shrinking response rate in Europe, which often drops below 50% and thus reduces the potential for generalizing findings. There is some evidence that those who do not respond to alcohol surveys are more likely to be either abstainers or heavy drinkers. Moreover, in many cultures, questions about alcohol may be perceived as stigmatizing, and under-reporting is a common problem. On the other hand, school surveys may be biased by both under- and over-reporting, as some youngsters tend to exaggerate their experiences associated with adulthood, including sexual ones as well as drinking and drug-taking.

Large health surveys which include only a few questions on alcohol also have serious disadvantages. As alcohol questions are considered sensitive, large surveys tend to offer these questions for self-administration which is very likely to produce errors, inconsistent responses or no response at all. Moreover, due to the prevailing public health paradigm, interest in such surveys may be reduced to frequent or heavy drinkers, which leads to the experience of light drinkers or abstainers being ignored.

European resources for monitoring

Common indicators and standardized data collection are essential for monitoring and evaluating national policies against a background of trends and developments in other countries and for sharing experiences in alcohol policy. European databases and surveys provide reference points for developing data collection and indicators at national level.

WHO's Global Information System on Alcohol and Health (GISAH) is the primary point of reference for tools for monitoring the health situation and trends in alcohol consumption, alcohol-related harm and policy responses (WHO, 2012). The regional sub-sections, such as the European Information System on Alcohol and Health (EISAH) maintained by the WHO Regional Office for Europe (WHO Regional Office for Europe, 2011b), provide region-specific information and enable comparisons at regional level. Alcohol-related data are organized in six main categories: levels of consumption; patterns of consumption; harms and consequences; economic aspects; alcohol control policies; and prevention, research and treatment. For example, the category alcohol-related harms and consequences includes statistics on alcohol-related morbidity and disease mortality as well as age-standardized death rates and DALYs for a range of health conditions, road traffic accidents and violence. The EISAH (which is still under development) will include tools for comparative risk assessment.

The data in the WHO alcohol and health information systems are updated through surveys addressed to Member States. Sources of complementary information include the burden of disease project as well as national studies and surveys. Alcohol consumption figures are based on official data on recorded adult per capita consumption supplied by Member States, complemented by data from economic operators and from the United Nation's Food and Agriculture Organization. As well as being used to update the online databases, the data collected are presented in status reports, such as the *European status report on alcohol and health* (WHO Regional Office for Europe, 2010) which includes country profiles comprising concise information on core indicators.

In recent years there has been increased collaboration between the EC and WHO in the development of data collection and health information systems, notably since 2007 in monitoring the trends in alcohol consumption, alcohol-related harm and alcohol-related policies across the EU. To complement the regular WHO surveys on alcohol and health, additional surveys and questions have been sent to EU member states. The data gathered are presented online in the European Union Information System on Alcohol and Health (EUSAH), maintained by WHO, which enables queries to be focused specifically on EU member states (European Commission, 2011). The information presented in the next chapter on the *EU status report on alcohol consumption, health outcomes and policies* was gathered in 2011 by means of a joint survey between the EC and the Regional Office.

To foster the collection of comparable data on health and health-related behaviour, diseases and health systems, the EC has developed the European Community Health Indicators (ECHI), which at the moment comprise 40 core indicators that are reasonably comparable and for which there is EU-wide agreement regarding definitions and data collection (European Commission, 2012a). Total alcohol consumption is included as a key determinant of health, measured by the consumption of pure alcohol per person aged 15 years and older. The information is provided by WHO.

The EC collects data on individual alcohol consumption through the European Health Interview Survey (EHIS), managed by Eurostat (EHIS, 2011). Starting from 2014, the EHIS will be conducted every five years in all EU member states. The survey includes a limited number of questions on the frequency and volume of alcohol consumption but does not measure health outcomes or other adverse consequences.

At the moment, EU-wide survey data on the drinking patterns of adults are only available in Eurobarometer surveys. The Eurobarometer is basically a public opinion survey tool. The surveys are carried out in all member states as face-to-face interviews, typically with representative samples of 600–1500 respondents aged 15 years and older (European Commission, 2012b). Alcohol-related data were gathered through Eurobarometer surveys on an ad hoc basis in 2006 and 2009.[10]

Alcohol consumption by teenagers is regularly monitored across Europe through two surveys. The Health Behaviour in School-Aged Children (HBSC) is a WHO collaborative cross-national study carried out at four-year intervals in practically all EU member states. The HSBC respondents are aged 11, 13 and 15 years (HBSC, 2002).[11] ESPAD is a collaborative initiative of international research teams, supported by the Council of Europe, the EC and the Swedish government. The ESPAD study is carried out every four years with the participation of almost all

---

[10] Examples are: *Attitudes towards alcohol*, Special Eurobarometer 272b/2007; and *EU citizens' attitudes towards alcohol*, Special Eurobarometer 331/2010. Questions relating to alcohol have also been included in surveys focused on other topics, for example: *Road safety*, Flash Eurobarometer 301/2010; and *Youth attitudes on drugs*, Flash Eurobarometer 330/2011 (European Commission, 2012b).

[11] The results of the 2009/2010 survey round are not yet available.

EU member states. The ESPAD respondents are schoolchildren aged 15–16 years (Hibell et al., 2009).[12] The HBSC and the ESPAD surveys are both carried out in a standardized fashion in order to produce comparable data for monitoring trends over time and enabling cross-country comparisons. Both surveys cover lifetime alcohol use, frequency of current use and drinking to drunkenness, using slightly different questions. The ESPAD survey also yields information on the volume of alcohol consumption as well as on risk perceptions and any harm experienced.

Along with national population surveys, the ESPAD survey is the main information source for reports from the European Monitoring Centre for Drugs and Drug Addiction (EMCDDA) in which alcohol consumption is examined along with illicit drugs, typically in a polydrug use context, and the data are used in annual reports on the state of the drugs problem in Europe or in reports focused on specific issues. An example is the selected issue report on *Drug use and related problems among very young people (under 15 years old)* (EMCDDA, 2007).

The variations in survey methods and a lack of comparable data on alcohol consumption patterns, which hamper cross-country comparisons and the forming of an overall view of alcohol consumption in the EU, were addressed in the EU-funded project on Standardizing Measurement of Alcohol Related Troubles (SMART) (SMART, 2012). The project collated and assessed the survey instruments for drinking habits used at national level in EU member states and developed a questionnaire which was pilot-tested in 10 member states with a total of 2000 respondents. The questionnaire proved to work well in the context of different drinking cultures, taking no more than 15–20 minutes in a face-to-face interview (Moskalewicz & Sierosławski, 2010). The final result is a standardized comparative survey methodology comprising the survey instrument and guidelines for application and for calculating annual alcohol consumption, unrecorded consumption, prevalence of episodic heavy drinking, prevalence of alcohol dependence, and alcohol-related harm for drinkers and for third parties. The survey instrument is currently available in 11 languages.

To facilitate the monitoring and assessment of progress towards the aims of the EU strategy to support member states in reducing alcohol-related harm (European Commission, 2006), the EC set up a Committee on Alcohol Data Collection, Indicators and Definitions, with the remit to identify common indicators for use at national and EU level based on existing sources of comparable data (European Commission, 2012c). The Committee identified three key indicators which they recommend for monitoring alcohol consumption and related harm:

- *volume of consumption* measured by total (recorded and unrecorded) yearly consumption of pure alcohol per capita (at age 15 years or older);
- *pattern of consumption* measured by harmful drinking defined as an intake of 60 g of pure alcohol or more on one occasion, monthly or more often, during the previous 12 months;
- *alcohol-attributable health harm* measured by alcohol-attributable years of life lost, with chronic and acute conditions as sub-indicators.

The source of information for the volume of alcohol consumption is the WHO alcohol information system. The source of information for harmful alcohol consumption (self-reported) will be the EHIS. Calculations relating to alcohol-attributable years of life lost can be done based on mortality statistics collected by Eurostat.

---

[12] The results of the 2011 survey round are not yet available.

Four indicators for monitoring trends in alcohol use among young people were selected from among the ESPAD survey items:

- *off-premise accessibility of alcohol*, measured by frequency of buying alcohol within the previous 30 days;
- *on-premise accessibility of alcohol*, measured by frequency of drinking on-premise within the previous 30 days;
- *binge-drinking*, defined as having five or more drinks on one or more occasions within the previous 30 days;[13]
- *prevalence of alcohol consumption by adolescents*, measured by the percentage of adolescents who report having drunk within the previous 12 months.

Three indicators were identified for monitoring trends in alcohol-related harm among adults, based on hospital discharge data and mortality data collected by Eurostat:

- *prevalence of alcohol-attributable chronic physical disorders*, measured by hospital discharge rates for alcoholic liver cirrhosis (ICD-10 code K70) and pancreatitis (ICD-10 codes K85–87) as proxy for alcohol-attributable disease;
- *prevalence of alcohol-attributable chronic mental disorders*, measured by hospital discharge rates;
- *alcohol-attributable death rates*.

Conclusions for policy and practice

Recent years have witnessed a substantial increase in the collection of data on alcohol consumption and alcohol-related harm across Europe and in work to strengthen the common knowledge base, including through initiatives by the EU, WHO and the OECD. This indicates wide recognition of the risks associated with alcohol use for individuals and society, and for health, welfare and economic development. The data collected at international level may overlap due to the use of the same original data sources. On the other hand, the same data may be provided in a slightly different form in response to subsequent requests. Further coordination at the international level would be needed to seek synergy so as to reduce the workload for national information providers and to increase comparability. Agreement would be crucial on common definitions of key indicators and on the manner of their presentation, including alcohol consumption data and vital statistics relating to health outcomes as well as economic and social harm and their costs.

Recent decades have also witnessed a proliferation of alcohol surveys in almost all EU countries as well as at EU level. The findings from these surveys are, for the most part, not comparable due to lack of standardized methodology. The two school surveys (HBSC and ESPAD) are an exception as they are carried out in all participating countries using the same methodology. The challenge is, however, that there is overlap in the targeted age groups and in the behaviour surveyed, including drinking by adolescents. Coordination would be needed to increase comparability, to reduce costs and to avoid situations where countries have to choose which survey they can afford to participate in.

---

[13] In the ESPAD survey instrument, a drink is defined as: approximately a glass/bottle/can of beer (25–33 cl), a glass/bottle/can of cider (25–33 cl), a bottle of alcopops (27 cl), a glass of wine (10–12.5 cl) or a glass of spirits (4 cl).

Perpetuating the *status quo* in this field, that is, spending resources on hundreds of national alcohol surveys which offer limited scope for international comparisons, is neither cost–effective nor helpful for monitoring progress towards common aims such as those of the EU strategy to support member states in reducing alcohol-related harm. A move towards the use of common instruments, such as the questionnaire developed in the SMART project, would be crucial for methodological advance and would, over time, reduce the costs of monitoring at both national and international level. An EU-wide or European drinking survey to gather comparable baseline information would be a necessary first step to encourage Member States to adopt common methodology.

The advantages of improved comparability are not limited to facilitating the monitoring of European strategies or action plans or to strengthening the methodological basis of national monitoring systems. The existence of comparable data and common indicators enables a discussion to take place of the merits and potential of the varying national alcohol policy approaches, helps avoid objectives which are not easily measurable, and may contribute to convergence across member states in public health policies to reduce alcohol-related harm.

References

European Commission (2006). *Communication from the Commission of 24 October 2006. An EU strategy to support Member States in reducing alcohol-related harm*. Brussels, European Commission (COM(2006) 625 final).

European Commission (2011). European Union Information System on Alcohol and Health (EUSAH) [web site]. Brussels, European Commission, Directorate-General Health & Consumers (http://ec.europa.eu/health/alcohol/policy/index_en.htm, accessed 29 February 2012).

European Commission (2012a). European Community Health Indicators (ECHI) [web site]. Brussels, European Commission, Directorate-General Health & Consumers (http://ec.europa.eu/health/indicators/echi/index_en.htm, accessed 29 February 2012).

European Commission (2012b). Eurobarometer surveys [web site]. Brussels, European Commission, Directorate-General Health & Consumers (http://ec.europa.eu/public_opinion/description_en.htm, accessed 29 February 2012).

European Commission (2012c). Alcohol-related indicators. Report on the work of the Committee on Alcohol Data, Indicators and Definitions [web site]. Brussels, European Commission (http://ec.europa.eu/health/indicators/committees/index_en.htm, accessed 29 February 2012).

EHIS (2011). *Glossary: European Health Interview Survey (EHIS)*. Brussels, European Commission (http://epp.eurostat.ec.europa.eu/statistics_explained/index.php/Glossary:European_health_interview_survey_%28EHIS%29, accessed 14 February 2012).

EMCDDA (2007). *Drug use and related problems among very young people (under 15 years old)*. Lisbon, European Monitoring Centre for Drugs and Drug Addiction (http://www.emcdda.europa.eu/attachements.cfm/att_44741_EN_TDSI07001ENC.pdf, accessed 29 February 2012) (Selected issue report).

EMCDDA (2012). European Monitoring Centre for Drugs and Drug Addiction [web site]. Lisbon, European Monitoring Centre for Drugs and Drug Addiction (http://www.emcdda.europa.eu/, accessed 29 February 2012).

ESPAD (2011). European School Survey Project on Alcohol and Other Drugs [web site]. Stockholm, The Swedish Council for Information on Alcohol and Other Drugs (http://www.espad.org/, accessed 29 February 2012).

Gordon R, Anderson P (2011). Science and alcohol policy: a case study of the EU strategy on alcohol. *Addiction,* 106(Suppl. 1):55–66.

HBSC (2002). Health Behaviour in School-aged Children: a World Health Organization cross-national study [web site]. St Andrews, Child and Adolescent Health Research Unit, University of St Andrews (http://www.hbsc.org, accessed 29 February 2012).

Hibbel B et al. (2009). *The 2007 ESPAD report. Substance use among students in 35 European countries.* Stockholm, CAN.

Karlsson T, Österberg E (2007). Scaling alcohol control policies across Europe. *Drugs: Education, Prevention, Policy*, 14(6):499–511.

Moskalewicz J, Sierosławski J (2010). *Drinking population surveys – guidance document for standardized approach. Final report prepared for the project Standardizing Measurement of Alcohol-Related Trouble – SMART.* Warsaw, Institute of Psychiatry and Neurology.

SMART (2012). Standardizing measurement of alcohol-related troubles (project SMART) [web site]. Warsaw, Institute of Psychiatry and Neurology (http://www.alcsmart.ipin.edu.pl/, accessed 14 February 2012).

WHO (2012). Global Information System on Alcohol and Health (GISAH) [web site]. Geneva, World Health Organization (http://www.who.int/gho/alcohol/en/index.html, accessed 29 February 2012).

WHO Regional Office for Europe (2010). *European status report on alcohol and health 2010.* Copenhagen, WHO Regional Office for Europe.

WHO Regional Office for Europe (2011a). *European Alcohol Action Plan to Reduce Harmful Use of Alcohol 2012–2020.* Copenhagen, WHO Regional Office for Europe.

WHO Regional Office for Europe (2011b). European Information System on Alcohol and Health (EISAH) [web site]. Copenhagen, WHO Regional Office for Europe (http://www.who.int/gho/alcohol/en/index.html, accessed 29 February 2012).

EU status report on public health policies on alcohol 2011

Julie Brummer and Lis Sevestre

Introduction

Since 2007, the EC and the Regional Office have joined forces in gathering information on trends in alcohol consumption, health outcomes and public health policies to reduce alcohol-related harms. In 2008, a survey on alcohol and health was for the first time carried out jointly by the EC and WHO. Carrying out joint surveys reduces the burden of reporting for member states and ensures the consistency and comparability of data across countries and over time.

This chapter reports the results of a second joint EC/WHO survey, carried out in May 2011. The survey was addressed to WHO national counterparts and to the national representatives in the EU Committee on Alcohol Policy and Action (CNAPA) (in some cases the same person fills both roles). The information reported here describes the situation as at 31 December 2010 (unless otherwise indicated). The survey covered all EU member states as well as Norway and Switzerland, which are members of the European Economic Area and regular participants in meetings of the CNAPA. With a 100% response rate from EU member states plus Norway and Switzerland, the information reported below covers 29 countries. The survey was also addressed to EU candidate countries in order to gather baseline information but, with the exception of key figures on alcohol consumption (Annexes 1 and 2), the data gathered are not reported here. The results relating to alcohol consumption and health outcomes are reported elsewhere in this volume (see the chapter on "Societal burden of alcohol").

Policy development at national level

Four out of five countries (23) reported the existence of a written national alcohol policy at the end of 2010. Since the previous survey in 2008,[14] three additional EU member states had adopted a written national alcohol policy. In addition, in 2011, one member state was in the process of drafting a national alcohol strategy.

Most respondents considered the elements of their respective national alcohol policies to have become stronger over the five years since 2006, set as the reference year because of the launch of the EU strategy to support member states in reducing alcohol-related harm (European Commission, 2006). Respondents were asked to rate given policy areas on a scale from minus 3 (weaker) to plus 3 (stronger). For the purposes of this analysis, responses were grouped in three categories, stronger, weaker and unchanged, and are summarized in Fig. 22.

Apart from drink–driving policies, for which 23 countries reported stronger developments, the two main areas where the greatest movement towards stronger policies occurred were public awareness-raising (22 countries) and community action (21 countries). The exceptions to the trend towards stronger policies were regulation of marketing, in which 17 countries reported no change and 3 weaker policies, and the affordability of alcohol, in which 13 countries reported no change and 3 weaker policies.

---

[14] 2008/2009 survey data were not available for Luxembourg and Greece.

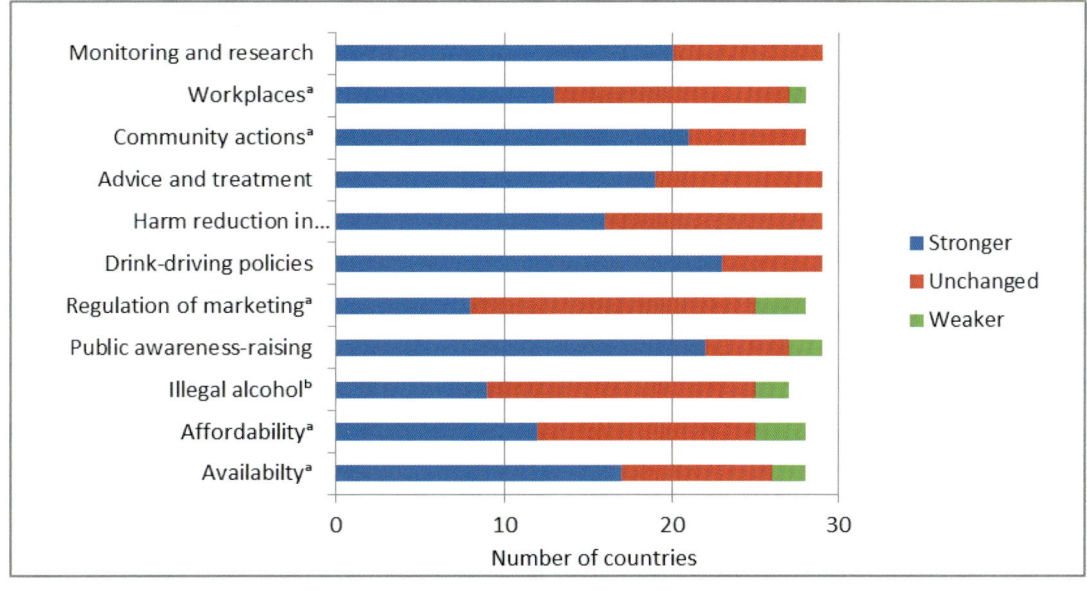

Fig. 22. Changes in alcohol policy areas over the five years since 2006 (N=29)

[a] Data missing from one country.
[b] Data missing from two countries.

Policies to address illegal alcohol were also an exception to the overall trend in the development of alcohol policies. Illegal alcohol may refer to illegally-produced or smuggled alcohol or the illegal sale of legally home-made (informally-produced) alcoholic beverages. Policies in this area, which may have varying importance in different countries, had mostly remained unchanged since 2006.

At the end of 2010, 26 countries reported having national rules to prevent the illegal production and sale of alcoholic beverages (Table 13). In 11 of the 26 countries (42%), the rules were enforced through administrative measures as opposed to criminal law. The use of duty-paid, excise or tax stamps or labels on alcoholic beverage containers/bottles was reported in 15 countries.

Table 13. Prevention of illegal production and sale of home- or informally-produced alcoholic beverages, end 2010

Rules and enforcement	No. of countries (N=29)
National rules to prevent illegal production and sale of home- or informally-produced alcoholic beverages[a]	26
Enforcement of rules through criminal law:[b]	
prison	6
fines	6
prison/fines	13
Enforcement of rules through other administrative measures	11

[a] Data missing from one country.
[b] Two countries did not have national rules.

In more than half of the countries (17), a comprehensive report on the alcohol situation in the country was regularly published. The range of topics covered varied considerably (Table 15).

Alcohol-related traffic accidents, harm to health and policy responses were among the most commonly monitored topics. As regards drinking habits, under-age drinking appeared to be monitored more closely than drinking by adults. Nevertheless, data on the rates of abstainers in the general population (Annex 2) as well as data on the rates of heavy episodic drinking (binge-drinking) among adults (Annex 3) were collected, at least sporadically, through national surveys in 27 of the 29 countries.

Table 15. Topics covered in regular published reports on alcohol situation

Topic	No. of countries (N=17)
Under-age drinking	12
Drinking among adults	6
Associations with socioeconomic variables	10
Geographical patterns of alcohol consumption	7
Associations with other substance use	5
Knowledge among the general public relating to alcohol	6
Drinking and pregnancy	4
Brief interventions within primary health care system	5
Alcohol-related hospital admissions/discharge data	11
Alcohol-attributable deaths	10
Drink–driving and alcohol-related traffic accidents	14
Alcohol-related public disorder and crime	6
Expenditure on alcohol-related harm	4
Affordability of alcohol	6
Availability of alcohol	7
Policy response	10

Price and tax measures

In the majority of countries an increase in the price of spirits (59%) and beer (62%), but not wine (48%), was reported relative to the consumer price index over the five years 2006–2010 (Fig. 23). What is not known is whether alcohol became more or less affordable during this time, taking into account changes in income. For the period 1966–2004, it is known that alcohol became more affordable in all EU member states, with the exception of Italy (Rabinovich et al., 2009).

Fig. 23. Trends in price of beer, wine and spirits relative to the consumer price index, previous five years (N=29), 2010

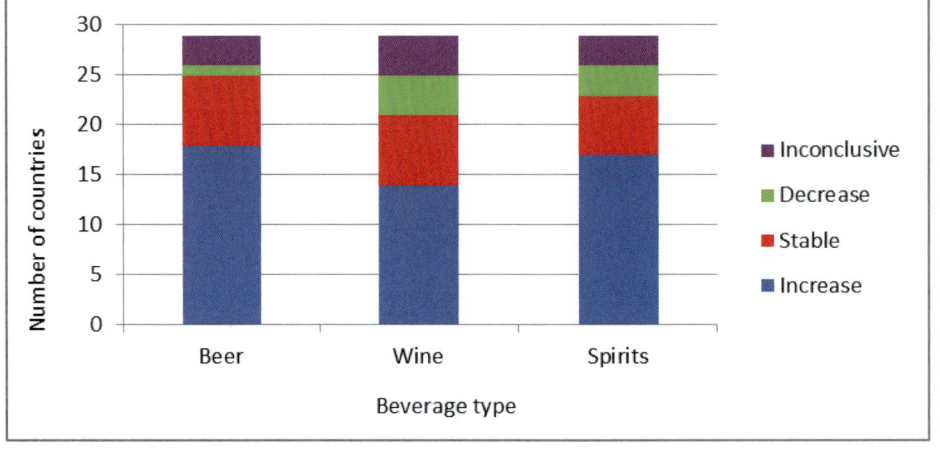

All countries levy excise duty on beer and spirits, but in eight countries wine is still not subject to this duty. Value added tax is levied on all alcoholic beverages (including wine) in all countries but, as with excise duty rates, its rates vary between beverage categories. Excise duties on alcoholic beverages are adjusted for inflation in only four countries.

As indicated in Table 16, other price measures implemented include an additional levy on specific products (alcopops and other ready-to-drink mixtures) (European Commission, 2009), a requirement to offer non-alcoholic beverages at a lower price than alcoholic beverages, and bans on volume discounts or below cost selling.

Table 16. Price and tax measures

Price and tax measures	No. of countries (N=29)
Excise duty on alcoholic beverages	29
beer	29
wine	21
spirits	29
alcoholic beverages, adjusted for inflation	4
Value added tax on alcoholic beverages	29
Imposition of minimum pricing	0
Ban on below-cost selling	1
Ban on volume discounts	2
Additional levy on specific products	5
Requirement to offer non-alcoholic beverages at a lower price	5

Availability of alcoholic beverages

Around two thirds of the countries require a licence for on- or off-premise sales but in 10 countries no licence is required (Table 17). In Finland, Norway and Sweden, alcoholic beverages above a given strength are sold through government-controlled retail monopolies.

Table 17. Countries requiring licensing (N=29), end 2010

	Beer	Wine	Spirits
Licences required for:			
on-premise sales	18[a]	19[a]	19[a]
off-premise sales	16[a]	17[a]	18[a]
Government monopolies of off-premise sales	3	3	3

[a]Data missing from two countries.

Almost all countries prohibit the sale of alcoholic beverages to intoxicated persons, and half or more restrict the places where sales are allowed or restrict sales at specific events. Only one third restrict the sale of alcoholic beverages in petrol stations and only a few countries reported restrictions on the times of sale or the density of outlets (Table 18).

All countries have set a legal minimum age limit for the on-premise sale of alcohol, and all but one (Italy) have a minimum age limit for off-premise sales as well. The most common minimum

Table 18. No. of countries with restrictions on on- and off-premise alcohol sales (N=29), end 2010

Restrictions	On-premise sales			Off-premise sales		
	Beer	Wine	Spirits	Beer	Wine	Spirits
Restrictions on hours	9	9	9	11	11	13
Restrictions on days	3	3	3	6	7	8
Restrictions on places	15	15	15	16	16	17
Restrictions on density	4	4	4	3	4	4
Restrictions on sales at specific events	20	21	21	20	21	22
Prohibition of sales to intoxicated persons	25	25	25	11	11	12

age is 18 years, applied to on-premise sales of spirits in 23 countries and to on-premise sales of beer and wine in 19 countries (Fig. 24). For off-premise sales, the 18-year minimum age (or higher) is used for spirits in 21 countries, and for beer and wine in 19 countries (Fig. 25). The beverage-specific age limits for each country as at the end of 2010 are listed in Table 19.

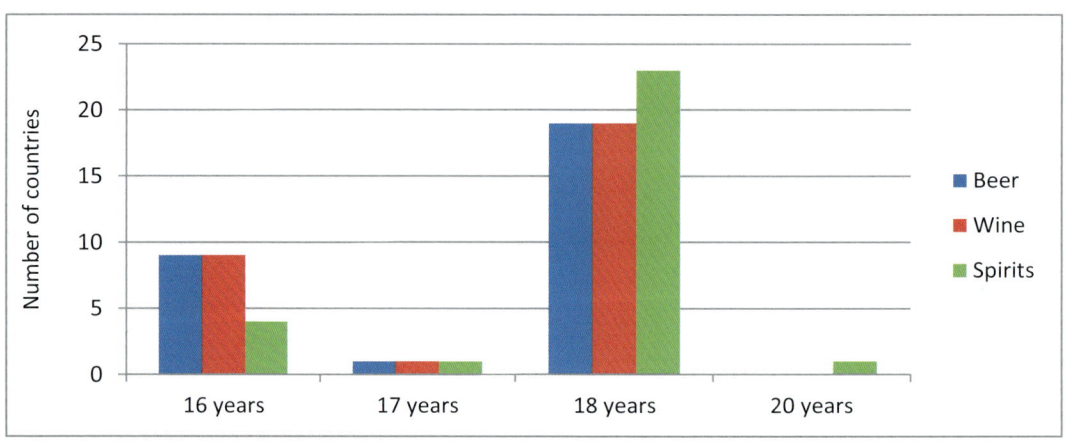

Fig. 24. Minimum age limits for on-premise sale of beer, wine and spirits, by number of countries (N=29), end 2010

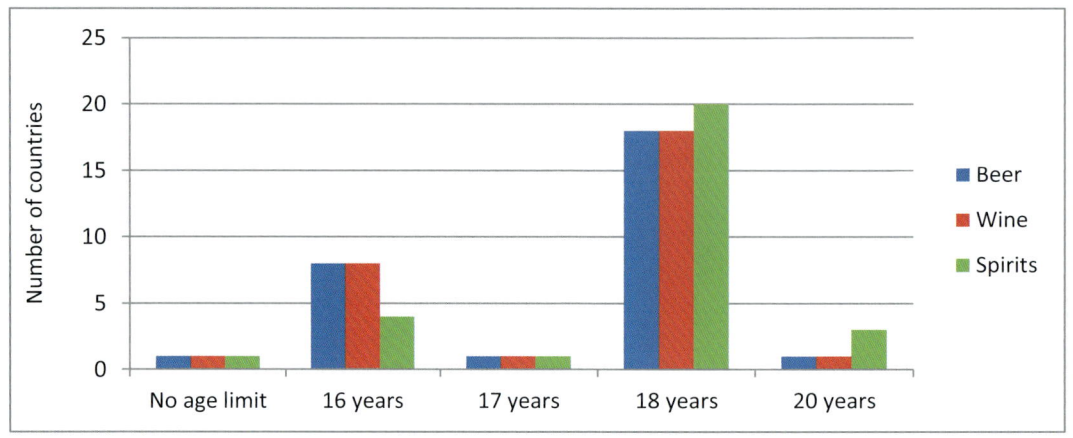

Fig. 25. Minimum age limits for off-premise sale of beer, wine and spirits, by number of countries (N=29), end 2010

Table 19. Minimum age limits for on-and off-premise sales of beer, wine and spirits, end 2010

Countries	On-premise sales			Off-premise sales		
	Beer	Wine	Spirits	Beer	Wine	Spirits
Austria	16	16	16	16	16	16
Belgium	16	16	18	16	16	18
Bulgaria	18	18	18	18	18	18
Cyprus	18	18	18	18	18	18
Czech Republic	18	18	18	18	18	18
Denmark	18	18	18	16	16	16[a]
Estonia	18	18	18	18	18	18
Finland	18	18	18	18	18	20
France	18	18	18	18	18	18
Greece	18	18	18	18	18	18
Germany	16	16	18	16	16	18
Hungary	18	18	18	18	18	18
Ireland	18	18	18	18	18	18
Italy	16	16	16	No age limit	No age limit	No age limit
Latvia	18	18	18	18	18	18
Lithuania	18	18	18	18	18	18
Luxembourg	16	16	16	16	16	16
Malta	17	17	17	17	17	17
Netherlands	16	16	18	16	16	18
Norway	18	18	20	18	18	20
Poland	18	18	18	18	18	18
Portugal	16	16	16	16	16	16
Romania	18	18	18	18	18	18
Slovakia	18	18	18	18	18	18
Slovenia	18	18	18	18	18	18
Spain	18	18	18	18	18	18
Sweden	18	18	18	20	20	20
Switzerland	16	16	18	16	16	18
United Kingdom	16	16	18	18	18	18

[a] On 7 March 2011, the age limit for buying alcohol products above 16.5% volume was raised to 18 years.

As regards the enforcement of age limits, respondents were asked to rate a range of possible measures in terms of importance in their countries, or indicate if the measure in question was not used at all (Table 20). Enforcement by the police or other authorities was rated as by far the most important measure, followed by awareness campaigns directed at sellers and servers or at young people.

Table 20. Importance of measures to enhance compliance with age limits, by number of countries (N=29), end 2010

Measures	High importance	Medium importance	Low importance	Not used at all
Server training on a voluntary basis	6	7	9	7
Server training as requirement of licensing system	8	7	3	11
Enforcement by the police or other authorities	17	10	2	0
Monitoring through test purchasing	7	12	3	7
Awareness campaigns directed at servers/sellers	10	6	7	6
Awareness campaigns directed at young people	10	13	4	2

In contrast, training for servers as a requirement linked with the serving licence or provided on a voluntary basis, as well as test purchasing (mystery shopping) to monitor compliance, were generally rated as having low importance or not used at all. Server training courses were, nevertheless, reported to be available nationwide in 17 countries, typically organized on a voluntary basis by businesses or trade associations (Table 21).

Table 21. No. of countries organizing training for servers, end 2010

Nationwide server training courses	No. of countries (N=29)
Organized on a regular basis	17
Organized on a voluntary basis by businesses or trade associations	10
Organized by trade/technical/vocational schools	5
Organized by enforcement agencies	1
Organized as a requirement of the national licensing system	5

A further aspect of the availability of alcoholic beverages covered in the survey concerned the emergence of new types of alcoholic beverage (Table 22). Spirits-based alcopops and ready-to-drink mixtures seem to be more or less established, reported in two thirds of the countries. Mixtures based on fermented alcohol (wine coolers, flavoured beers, flavoured ciders) were reported in one third or half of the countries. Alcoholic energy drinks or other high-caffeine drinks seem to be still emerging, reported in fewer than one third of the countries.

Table 22. New alcoholic beverages

Beverages	No. of countries (N=29)
New types of alcoholic beverage:	21
spirits-based mixtures/alcopops	18
alcopops based on fermented alcohol	11
wine coolers/wine-based mixtures	12
flavoured/designer beers	16
flavoured/designer ciders	12
alcoholic energy drinks	8
other high-caffeine alcoholic drinks	6
alcoholic gels or powders	1

Policies on the marketing of alcoholic beverages

Legally binding regulations on alcohol advertising are in place in 26 countries at national level and in one country at sub-national level. Only two countries reported that no regulations have been implemented through legislation. Altogether, 21 countries also have legally binding regulations on product placement, either at national (20) or sub-national level (1).

Restrictions on marketing, product placement and sponsorship were patchy at best with most countries having partial statutory restrictions, typically on broadcast or print advertising of alcoholic beverages, and many countries with no restrictions for many media. In this survey, information was not gathered on the young people's exposure to alcohol advertising, although the volume of exposure is the key ingredient for potential harm and the factor the restrictions are intended to address. Alcohol advertising on the internet is among the least regulated domains, despite the popularity of online media among young people and the importance of social media in influencing behaviour. The number of countries with regulations on the advertising of alcoholic beverages and product placement in different media are summarized in Tables 23–25 separately for beer, wine and spirits. Total bans on alcohol advertising are applied more often to broadcast media than to print media, and more often on spirits advertising than on the advertising of beer or wine.

Table 23. Countries with restrictions on advertising/product placement for beer, end 2010

Media	Total ban	Partial statutory restriction	Voluntary agreement/ self-regulation	No restriction
Advertising				
Public service/national TV	4	18	1	6
Commercial/private TV	3	19	1	6
National radio	3	18	2	6
Local radio	2	18	3	6
Printed newspapers/magazines	1	13	6	9
Billboards	2	12	5	10
Points of sale	1	10	5	13
Cinema	3	12	4	10
Internet	1	10	6	12
Product placement				
Public service/national TV	5	12	2	10
Commercial/private TV	4	12	2	11

Table 24. Countries with restrictions on advertising/product placement for wine, end 2010

Media	Total ban	Partial statutory restriction	Voluntary agreement/ self-regulation	No restriction
Advertising				
Public service/national TV	5	19	0	5
Commercial/private TV	4	20	0	5
National radio	4	19	1	5
Local radio	3	19	2	5
Printed newspapers/magazines	2	13	5	9
Billboards	3	12	4	10
Points of sale	1	11	4	13
Cinema	4	13	3	12
Internet	2	10	5	12
Product placement				
Public service/national TV	5	14	1	9
Commercial/private TV	4	14	1	10

Some three out of five countries reported that they had some form of national restriction on alcohol industry sponsorships or sales promotions. Table 26 summarizes the reported restrictions on industry sponsorships and sales promotions by beverage category. The restrictions, when in place, tended to be partial, with stronger restrictions reported for spirits. Depending on the beverage type and category of sponsorship/promotion, between 11 and 17 countries reported no restrictions.

Table 25. Countries with restrictions on advertising/product placement for spirits, end 2010

Media	Total ban	Partial statutory restriction	Voluntary agreement/ self-regulation	No restriction
Advertising				
Public service/national TV	10	15	1	3
Commercial/private TV	9	16	1	3
National radio	8	16	2	3
Local radio	7	16	3	3
Printed newspapers/magazines	4	10	6	9
Billboards	7	7	5	10
Points of sale	4	8	5	12
Cinema	7	10	4	8
Internet	6	6	6	11
Product placement				
Public service/national TV	6	13	2	8
Commercial/private TV	5	13	2	9

Table 26. Countries with restrictions on sponsorship and sales promotions

Sponsorships and sales promotions	Total ban	Partial statutory restriction	Voluntary agreement/ self-regulation	No restriction
Beer				
Industry sponsorship of sporting events	3	9	5	12
Industry sponsorship of youth events	4	8	5	12
Sales promotion from producers	2	9	3	15
Sales promotion from retailers (including supermarkets)	3	8	2	16
Sales promotion from owners of pubs and bars in the form of serving alcohol for free	4	6	2	17
Wine				
Industry sponsorship of sporting events	3	9	5	12
Industry sponsorship of youth events	4	8	5	12
Sales promotion from producers	3	8	3	15
Sales promotion from retailers (including supermarkets)	5	6	2	16
Sales promotion from owners of pubs and bars in the form of serving alcohol for free	4	6	2	17
Spirits				
Industry sponsorship of sporting events	7	7	4	11
Industry sponsorship of youth events	7	6	3	12
Sales promotion from producers	6	7	3	13
Sales promotion from retailers (including supermarkets)	6	6	2	15
Sales promotion from owners of pubs and bars in the form of serving alcohol for free	5	6	2	16

Information and education

As regards activities to reduce alcohol-related harm through awareness-raising, information and education, the survey covered policies relating to school-based education on alcohol, nationwide awareness-raising activities carried out during the previous three years, and the use of alcoholic beverage packages or alcohol advertisements as a vehicle for raising awareness about risks related to alcohol consumption.

Twenty countries (69%) reported that education programmes relating to alcohol (or broader substance use) are carried out nationwide as part of the school curriculum, in most cases as a legal requirement. National guidelines for the prevention and reduction of alcohol-related harm in school settings were available in 15 countries (Table 27).

Table 27. No. of countries with school-based education and policies, end 2010

Education and policies	No. of countries (N=29)
Nationwide educational programmes involving teachers, schoolchildren and/or parents as part of the school curriculum	20
Legal obligation for schools to carry out alcohol prevention as part of school curriculum/health policies	18
National guidelines for the prevention and reduction of alcohol-related harm in school settings	15

The survey also enquired about awareness-raising activities during the previous three years. As illustrated in Table 28, all countries carried out some form of national awareness-raising activity, with most addressing young people's drinking (83% of the countries) and drink–driving (93% of the countries) and, to a lesser extent, the impact of alcohol on health (72% of the countries).

Table 28. No. of countries with awareness-raising activities during previous three years, end 2010

Activities	No. of countries (N=29)
Some form of national awareness-raising activity	29
Activity:	
drinking by young people	24
drink–driving	27
indigenous people	1
impact of alcohol on health	21
social harms	12
illegal/surrogate alcohol	1
alcohol and pregnancy	14
alcohol at work	10

Nine countries had a legal requirement at national level for health warning labels to be placed on alcohol advertisements. Examples included: "Attention! This is an alcoholic product. Alcohol may harm your health!" (Estonia), "Alcohol abuse is harmful for your health" (France), and "Minister of Health warns: Alcohol consumption may damage your health!" (Slovenia).

In contrast, only two countries reported a legal requirement at national level to place health warning labels on alcoholic beverage containers. The warning in Portugal was "Drink in moderation".

Community action

All but two countries reported the presence of community-based intervention projects involving young people and/or civil society, with nongovernmental organizations and local government bodies as the most commonly involved stakeholders. Eleven countries reported the availability of national guidelines for implementing effective community-based interventions to reduce alcohol-related harm (Table 29).

Table 29. No. of countries with stakeholder involvement

Community action	No. of countries (N=29)
National guidelines for implementing effective community-based interventions to reduce alcohol-related harm	11
Community-based intervention projects involving any stakeholders:	27
nongovernmental organizations	26
economic operators	13
local government bodies	25
Interventions/projects actively involving young people/civil society	25

Health sector responses

Questions in the survey relating to the health services addressed the availability of a range of responses and services. Brief interventions for health promotion and disease prevention, counselling for pregnant women with alcohol use disorders or alcohol problems, and counselling for children in families with alcohol problems were reported as available in some three quarters of the countries (Table 30).

Table 30. No. of countries offering services and interventions by the health services

Services	No. of countries (N=29)
Overall health services response	
Brief interventions for health promotion and disease prevention	21
Training of health professionals in screening and brief interventions for alcohol problems	14
Clinical guidelines for brief interventions endorsed by at least one health care professional body	18
Obstetric and pregnancy care	
Counselling for pregnant women with alcohol use disorders or alcohol problems	21
Prenatal care services to pregnant women with alcohol use disorders or alcohol problems	15
Services for children and family members	
Counselling for children in families with alcohol problems	22

Alcohol and the workplace

A set of questions addressed the prevention of alcohol-related harm in workplace settings. Eighteen countries reported that prevention or counselling programmes were available at workplaces, although national guidelines for workplace activities were only available in eight countries. In 10 countries, testing for alcohol or drugs at workplaces was governed by legislation.

In 11 countries social partners representing employers and employees were involved at national level in action to prevent and address alcohol-related harm at workplaces (Table 31).

Table 31. No. of countries with workplace services and prevention, end 2010

Workplace services and legislation	No. of countries (N=29)
Prevention or counselling programmes at workplaces	18
National guidelines for prevention of and counselling for alcohol problems at workplaces	8
Involvement of social partners representing employers and employees in action to prevent and address alcohol-related harm at workplaces	11
Legislation on alcohol testing at workplaces	10[a]

[a] Data missing from one country.

Alcohol-free environments

Most countries reported that they had prohibitions or restrictions on the consumption of alcoholic beverages in public places, usually in educational buildings, on public transport, at sporting events and in health care establishments. Half the countries also prohibited or restricted drinking in workplaces, government offices and outdoor environments (parks, streets, etc.) (Table 32).

Table 32. No. of countries with restrictions on alcohol consumption in public venues (N=29), end 2010

Public venues	Statutory ban or restrictions	Voluntary agreement/ self-regulation	No restriction
Health care establishments	16	6	7
Educational buildings	18	7	4
Government offices	14	9	6
Public transport	17	6	6
Parks, streets, etc.	15	6	8
Sporting events	17	9	3
Leisure events	8	9	12
Workplaces	14	12	3
Places of religious worship[a]	5	12	11

[a] Data missing from one country.

Drink–driving countermeasures

At the end of 2010, all but three countries had established a maximum legal BAC level of 0.5 g/litre or below for general population drivers, with four countries adopting a zero tolerance level (Fig. 26). Towards the end of 2011, Ireland reduced its maximum permitted BAC level from 0.8 g/litre to 0.5 g/litre for general population drivers. This left only Malta and the United Kingdom with a level of 0.8 g/litre (Table 33). Figs. 27 and 28 show that at the end of 2010 lower maximum BAC levels were reported for novice and commercial drivers.

Breath-testing was widely used to enforce BAC limits, with at least half of the countries implementing random breath-testing either by mobile police patrol units or in stationary roadside checkpoints (Table 34).

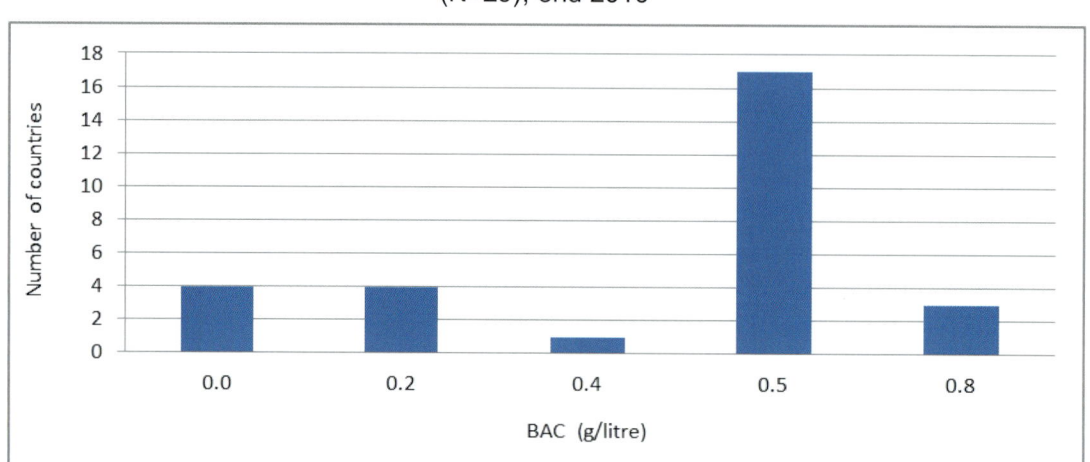

Fig. 26. Maximum legal BAC level for the general population, by number of countries (N=29), end 2010

Table 33. National maximum BAC levels (g/litre), end 2010

Countries	General population	Novice drivers	Commercial drivers
Austria	0.05	0.10	0.10
Belgium	0.05	0.05	0.05
Bulgaria	0.05	0.05	0.05
Cyprus	0.05	0.05	0.05
Czech Republic	0.00	0.00	0.00
Denmark	0.05	0.05	0.05
Estonia	0.02	0.02	0.02
Finland	0.05	0.05	0.05
France	0.05	0.05	0.02
Greece	0.05	0.02	0.02
Germany	0.05	0.00	0.00
Hungary	0.00	0.00	0.00
Ireland[a]	0.08	0.08	0.08
Italy	0.05	0.00	0.00
Latvia	0.05	0.02	0.05
Lithuania	0.04	0.02	0.02
Luxembourg	0.05	0.02	0.02
Malta	0.08	0.08	0.08
Netherlands	0.05	0.02	0.05
Norway	0.02	0.02	0.00
Poland	0.02	0.02	0.02
Portugal	0.05	0.05	0.05
Romania	0.00	0.00	0.00
Slovakia	0.00	0.00	0.00
Slovenia	0.05	0.00	0.00
Spain	0.05	0.03	0.03
Sweden	0.02	0.02	0.02
Switzerland	0.05	0.05	0.05
United Kingdom	0.08	0.08	0.08

Using a scale from 0 (not enforced) to 10 (fully enforced), respondents were asked to consider, at the national level, the level of enforcement of the maximum legal BAC for drivers. The results are summarized in Fig. 29. At the high end of the scale, one country rated the level of enforcement at 10 and 14 countries rated it at 8 or 9; the minimum reported level of enforcement was 4 in one country.

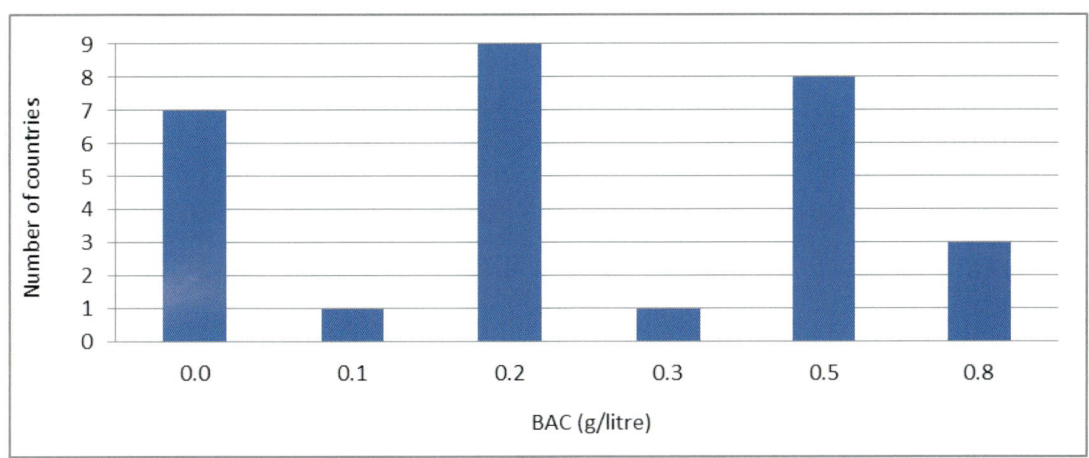

Fig 27. Maximum legal BAC level for novice drivers, by number of countries (N=29), end 2010

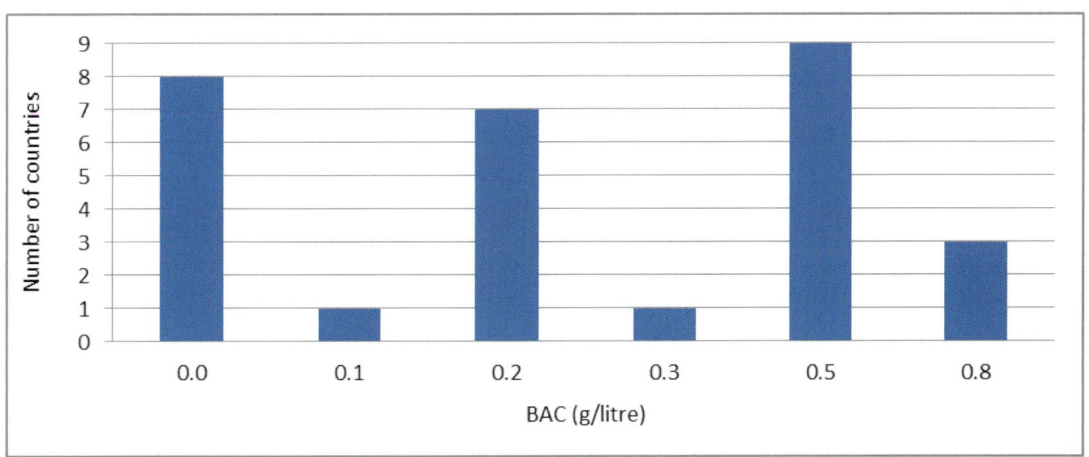

Fig. 28. Maximum legal BAC level for commercial drivers, by number of countries, (N=29), end 2010

Table 34. No. of countries enforcing maximum legal BAC, end 2010

Measures	No. of countries (N=29)
Random breath-testing at roadside stationary police checkpoints	16
Random breath-testing by special mobile patrol units	20
Selective breath-testing	19
Breath-testing of all drivers involved in a crash	19
Blood-testing of all drivers involved in a crash	10

As mentioned above, drink–driving was the most common topic in nationwide awareness-raising campaigns carried out during the previous three years. As regards the targeted prevention of drink–driving, 15 countries reported mandatory education or treatment programmes for habitual offenders. The use of alcohol ignition interlocks (devices which prevent the vehicle from starting unless the driver passes a breathalyser test) was reported in seven countries, usually in relation to commercial transport or with drink–driving offenders as an alternative to punishment (driving ban) in combination with rehabilitation (Table 35).

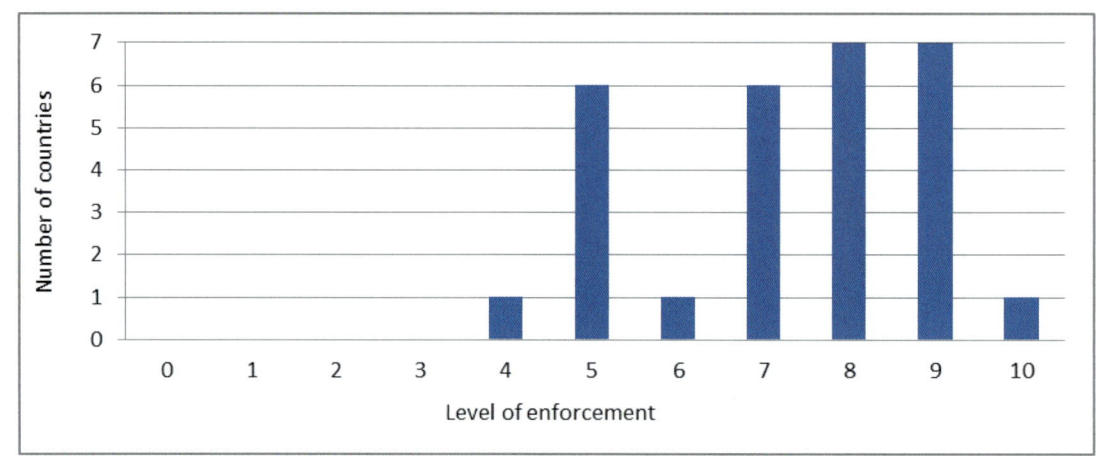

Fig. 29. Level of enforcement at national level (on scale from 0 to 10) of maximum legal BAC when driving a vehicle, by number of countries (N=29)

Table 35. Other drink–driving prevention strategies

Prevention strategy	No. of countries (N=29)
Mandatory driver education/treatment programmes for habitual offenders	15
Any use of alcolocks:	7
– in pilot projects	1
– in combination with rehabilitation as an alternative to punishment	4
– voluntary use by public or commercial transport companies	5
– obligatory use by public or commercial transport companies	2
– voluntary use by individual drivers	2

References

European Commission (2006). *Communication from the Commission of 24 October 2006. An EU strategy to support Member States in reducing alcohol-related harm*. Brussels, European Commission (COM(2006) 625 final).

European Commission (2009). *First progress report on the implementation of the EU alcohol strategy. Annex 1: Development of alcohol policy and action in EU Member States 2006–2009*. Brussels, European Commission, Directorate-General for Health and Consumers.

European Commission (2011). *Excise duty tables. Part I – Alcoholic beverages*. Brussels, European Commission, Directorate-General for Taxation and Customs Union (Ref 1.033).

Rabinovich L et al. (2009). *The affordability of alcohol beverages in the European Union: understanding the link between alcohol affordability, consumption and harms*. Cambridge, RAND Europe.

Conclusions

Peter Anderson and Lars Møller

This report shows us that we in Europe still face an enormous challenge to reduce the major health burden that alcohol places on Europe's citizens. For the EU as a whole, the level of per capita alcohol consumption (the main determinant of harm) did not change during the first decade of the 2000s and remains stuck at 12.5 litres of pure alcohol per year among the adult population (aged 15 years and over). This works out at an average of 27 g of pure alcohol – nearly three drinks – a day.

Alcohol diminishes our personal security. Alcohol is an intoxicant affecting a wide range of structures and processes in the central nervous system which, interacting with personality characteristics, associated behaviour and sociocultural expectations, is a causal factor for intentional and unintentional injuries and harm to people other than the drinker, including interpersonal violence, suicide, homicide, crime and drink–driving fatalities, and a causal factor for risky sexual behaviour, sexually transmitted diseases and HIV infection.

Alcohol impairs our health. Alcohol is a potent teratogen with a range of negative outcomes to the fetus, including low birth weight, cognitive deficiencies and fetal alcohol disorders. It is neurotoxic to brain development, leading in adolescence to structural hippocampal changes and, in middle age, to reduced brain volume. It is a dependence-producing drug, similar to other substances under international control, through its reinforcing properties and neuroadaptation in the brain. It is an immunosuppressant, increasing the risk of communicable diseases and their effective treatment, including tuberculosis, community-acquired pneumonia and HIV/AIDS. Alcoholic beverages and the ethanol in them are classified as a carcinogen by the International Agency for Research on Cancer, increasing the risk of cancers of the oral cavity and pharynx, oesophagus, stomach, colon, rectum and breast in a linear dose–response relationship. Alcohol is overwhelmingly detrimental to the cardiovascular system, being a cause of hypertension, haemorrhagic stroke and atrial fibrillation. Chronic heavy use increases the risk of ischaemic heart disease and stroke, whereas average light to moderate drinking decreases the risk, with this decreased risk wiped out by just one heavy drinking occasion a month. The real absolute risk of dying from alcohol increases simply and linearly with the total amount of alcohol consumed over a lifetime, such that at a consumption of 60 g of alcohol per day, the risk reaches 1 in 10.

Alcohol diminishes our human capital by interfering with educational attainment, increasing the both the risk of unemployment and absenteeism and presenteeism. At any given level of alcohol consumption, the more socially disadvantaged people are in terms of education or income, the more likely they are to suffer from alcohol-related harm and die from an alcohol-related condition.

No wonder, then, that in the population aged 25–59 years – often the core productive years – alcohol is the world's number one risk factor for impaired health and premature death, and far more significant than unsafe sex, tobacco use or diabetes. No wonder too, that in the EU, alcohol is the cause of 1 in 10 deaths among people aged 15–64 years.

Alcohol is not just a health issue; it is also a vital issue for the economy and for productivity. At times of economic downturns, the two conditions for which death rates jump up are suicides and alcohol use disorders. A more than 3% increase in unemployment in the EU is associated with a staggering 28% increase in deaths from alcohol use disorders. Many studies have estimated the economic burden that alcohol imposes on society. The cost comes to as much as 2–3% of GDP, over €300 per citizen per year; and between half and two thirds of these social costs are due to lost productivity. If the costs to people other than the drinker are included, this cost would probably double.

The EU faces an urgent need to reduce the burden of alcohol, not only to improve the health and well-being of its citizens but also to strengthen the economic sustainability and productivity of the Union as a whole.

Fortunately, as this volume reports, there are many effective and cost–effective ways to do this. Indeed, a joint report by the World Economic Forum and WHO for the September 2011 United Nations High Level meeting on noncommunicable diseases included three actions on alcohol (tax increases, restricted access to retail alcohol and bans on alcohol advertising) as being among the "best buys" to reduce the global burden of noncommunicable diseases (Bloom et al., 2011; WHO and World Economic Forum, 2011; WHO, 2011).

This volume has shown that increasing the *price of alcohol*, relative to other goods and incomes, is the key to reducing alcohol-related harm. There is an enormous wealth of evidence to show that this is a highly effective and cost–effective measure. Concern is sometimes expressed that price increases do not make any impact on heavier drinkers and unfairly penalize lighter drinkers. The evidence included in this report shows that this is simply not the case. Price increases have an increased differential impact on heavier drinkers, and reduce all types of alcohol-related harm. Lighter drinkers also suffer from alcohol-related harm, so, if they reduce their consumption subsequent to a price increase, they will also accrue benefit. Of course, tax increases are not necessarily followed through to price increases, and there is increasing evidence describing the extent to which producers and retailers absorb some or much of a tax increase. A policy option, much discussed at present, to get round this problem is to set a minimum price per gram of alcohol sold. This has been done for many years in parts of Canada, and it reduces harm. Modelling studies, at least those done for the United Kingdom (England and Scotland) robustly predict major health and economic benefits from the introduction of a minimum price per gram of alcohol.

This report has also shown that the *availability of alcohol and exposure to its marketing*, including through the social media and communication devices, have an impact on alcohol consumption and alcohol-related harm. The policy conclusions are obvious. Health benefit occurs from reducing the retail availability of alcohol and from reducing the volume of exposure to all forms of commercial communication about alcohol.

The volume shows that even though more and more alcohol is consumed outside *licensed premises*, what goes on inside those premises can have an impact on alcohol-related harm. Two important things stand out: the physical and social design of the premises, which can be designed to reduce drunkenness, and the correct incentives to sellers, backed up where necessary by legal enforcement, to promote less risky drinking rather than intoxication.

For people in work, what goes on in the *workplace* can reduce harm. In workplaces where stress is an important factor, the risk of alcohol use disorders and alcohol dependence is increased. Workplaces that embed alcohol programmes within wellness at work initiatives seem to reduce the negative consequences of alcohol.

Drink–driving policies are a special case of alcohol policy. The evidence is simple and straightforward. The lower the legal BAC for drinking and the stronger the implementation, the safer European roads will be.

No matter what kind of policy or programme is implemented, people are still going to get into trouble with alcohol by drinking too much or being defined as dependent on alcohol. Here, the evidence is clear that both *brief advice programmes* for people with risky drinking habits and *treatment programmes* for those with alcohol use disorders can make an enormous difference. The remaining problem, albeit a very large one, is implementation: the vast majority (somewhere between 90% and 95%) of those who could benefit from brief advice or treatment simply do not get offered them. This remains a great challenge to the health care sector.

This volume has shown that there are some policy options that do not work in isolation. Repeated evidence shows that *school-based programmes* do not materially reduce the harm done by alcohol among young people. This is hardly surprising given the huge amount of commercial communications, availability and cheapness of alcohol surrounding young people, especially when young people perceive themselves as singled out. Most alcohol harm and alcohol-related deaths in fact occur among their parents and middle-aged people. This is not to say that education is not important; rather it has to be part of and in support of the implementation of an effective and comprehensive policy.

Neither do *community programmes* work in isolation. Community programmes only work when they are implementing policies and action known to be effective, such as drink–driving countermeasures or the enforcement of laws about selling and serving. Again, this is not to say that community action is not important. It is important to implement policy at the local level, but it will only have an effect when it is based on known programmes and policies that do actually work in reducing alcohol-related harm.

To be effective, policy has to be *comprehensive* across the whole range of action. This was illustrated by the cost–effectiveness analyses where combined policies were more cost–effective in reducing alcohol-related harm than the simple addition of separate policies. It was also demonstrated by the ECAS data in the chapter on effectiveness and cost–effectiveness, which showed that, over time, the more comprehensive a policy is in a country, the lower is the alcohol consumption.

The basic message coming through this report is that if it is really desired to make a difference in reducing the harm done by alcohol, it will be necessary to implement what is known to work. So, finally, in this respect what progress is being made?

With regard to price, the majority of respondents to the WHO survey (summarized in the chapter on the WHO/EC survey on alcohol and health 2011) reported an increase in the price of spirits (59%) and beer (62%), but not wine (48%) relative to the consumer price index over the five years 2006–2010. What is not known is whether alcohol became more or less affordable during this time, accounting for changes in income. For the period 1966–2004, it is known that alcohol became more affordable in all EU member states studied, with the exception of Italy.

With regard to availability, 10 countries did not require a licence for the sale of alcohol and very few countries restricted the density of outlets or the times of sale. Nevertheless, all countries had a minimum age limit for the sale of alcohol on licensed premise, and all countries but one (Italy) had set a minimum age limit for off-premise purchases, the most common age being 18 years.

Restrictions on marketing, product placement and sponsorship were patchy at best, with most countries having partial statutory restrictions and many countries no restrictions for many media. Information was not available on the volume of exposure, which is the key ingredient for potential harm, or the use of social media, which is now regarded as the most influential media form for impacts on behaviour.

Fewer than two thirds of countries (62%) reported the existence of prevention or counselling programmes at workplaces. Unfortunately no information was available on the extent to which these are implemented across the workforce. Although the evidence suggests a limited impact, 17 countries (59%) reported that nationwide server training courses were organized on a regular basis.

All but two countries (Malta and the United Kingdom) reported a legal BAC level for driving of 0.5 g/litre or less. Twelve countries (41%) still had a legal level of 0.5 g/litre or more for commercial drivers. Twenty countries (69%) reported the implementation of random breath-testing by special police patrol units, although objective measures of enforcement were not known.

When it comes to health sector responses, 21 countries (72%) reported the availability of brief interventions for health promotion and disease prevention, and the same proportion for counselling to pregnant women with alcohol use disorders or alcohol problems. But, as mentioned above, the key issue here is the proportion of people in need who receive advice or counselling, and this tends to be as little as 5% or 10%.

Twenty countries (69%) reported the availability of nationwide school-based programmes and all countries had reported some type of awareness-raising activity implemented during the previous three years. Despite the fact that alcohol is a carcinogen, only two countries reported a legal requirement to place health warning labels on alcoholic beverage containers, with the stated messages unlikely to have much impact. All but two countries reported the presence of community-based intervention projects involving a range of stakeholders.

Four out of five countries (23) reported the existence of a written national alcohol policy. Most countries considered that the elements of alcohol policies had become stronger over the five years since 2006. Apart from drink–driving policies, in which 23 countries reported stronger developments, the two main areas with the greatest development for stronger policies were public awareness-raising (22 countries) and community action (21 countries). The two main exceptions to stronger policies were regulation of marketing, in which 17 countries reported no change and 3 weaker policies, and the affordability of alcohol, in which 13 countries had reported no change and 3 weaker policies. Finally, two fifths of countries (12) did not regularly publish a comprehensive report on the alcohol situation in the country.

To sum up, over the past five years the policies that have got stronger, such as awareness-raising and community action, are not part of WHO's best buys, whereas the policies that have tended not to get stronger, such as affordability of alcohol and regulating of marketing, are part of WHO's best buys. There is thus a great opportunity to reduce the burden of alcohol on individuals and societies, as well as on the EU as a whole, over the coming years.

References

Bloom DE et al. (2011). *The global economic burden of non-communicable diseases*. Geneva, World Economic Forum.

WHO (2011). *Global status report on noncommunicable diseases 2010*. Geneva, World Health Organization (http://www.who.int/nmh/publications/ncd_report_full_en.pdf, accessed 24 February 2012).

WHO and World Economic Forum (2011). *From burden to "best buys": reducing the economic impact of non-communicable diseases in low- and middle-income countries*. Geneva, World Economic Forum (http://www.who.int/nmh/publications/best_buys_summary.pdf, accessed 24 February 2012).

Annex 1

ADULT PER CAPITA ALCOHOL CONSUMPTION IN THE EU, CANDIDATE COUNTRIES, NORWAY AND SWITZERLAND (2009)

Country	Total consumption (litres)	Unrecorded (litres)
Austria	13.00	0.7
Belgium	12.00	1.0
Bulgaria	11.45	1.2
Croatia	12.76	2.5
Cyprus	9.53	1.0
Czech Republic	16.61	1.5
Denmark	12.86	2.0
Estonia	14.05	0.7
Finland	12.27	2.3
France	12.70	0.4
Germany	12.87	1.0
Greece	10.55	1.8
Hungary	14.15	2.5
Iceland[a]	7.93	0.4
Ireland	12.87	1.0
Italy	9.59	2.4
Latvia	Under review	
Lithuania	13.02	0.4
Luxembourg	12.76	1.0
The former Yugoslav Republic of Macedonia	6.84	2.9
Malta[a]	8.01	0.4
Montenegro	13.02	4.7
Netherlands	9.73	0.5
Norway[a]	8.30	1.6
Poland	13.60	3.0
Portugal	13.43	2.0
Romania[b]	16.30	3.0
Slovakia	14.59	3.0
Slovenia	15.31	3.0
Spain	13.07	1.4
Sweden	8.85	1.7
Switzerland	10.76	0.5
Turkey	3.64	2.2
United Kingdom	12.52	1.7
EU	12.45	1.6

[a] Adult per capita consumption of alcohol equal to or less than 70% of the EU average.
[b] Adult per capita consumption of alcohol equal to or greater than 130% of the EU average.

Annex 2

LIFETIME ABSTAINERS IN THE EU, CANDIDATE COUNTRIES, NORWAY AND SWITZERLAND BY COUNTRY AND GENDER (2009)

Country	Lifetime abstainers, men (%)	Lifetime abstainers, women (%)
Austria	4.80	8.50
Belgium	3.40	12.50
Bulgaria	8.50	31.50
Croatia	11.70	31.31
Cyprus	6.40	13.70
Czech Republic	2.80	6.30
Denmark	0.60	0.90
Estonia	7.40	13.60
Finland	3.30	10.50
France	1.80	3.30
Germany	1.30	2.00
Greece	6.70	21.00
Hungary	3.60	9.40
Iceland	5.10	12.80
Ireland	16.70	24.30
Italy	5.80	19.40
Latvia	5.70	13.80
Lithuania	4.30	16.60
Luxembourg	5.90	14.80
The former Yugoslav Republic of Macedonia	29.46	51.50
Malta	6.20	14.60
Montenegro	11.70	31.31
Netherlands	6.10	16.70
Norway	2.30	4.10
Poland	6.80	20.90
Portugal	18.60	32.00
Romania	6.50	19.10
Slovakia	7.40	7.10
Slovenia	3.70	8.90
Spain	9.50	24.70
Sweden	5.30	10.80
Switzerland	7.30	20.60
Turkey	64.97	91.88
United Kingdom	8.90	15.20
Total EU	**5.60**	**13.50**

Annex 3

RATES OF HEAVY EPISODIC DRINKING (BINGE-DRINKING)

Country	National surveys on rates of heavy episodic drinking	Heavy episodic drinking among males (%)	Heavy episodic drinking among females (%)	Year of survey	Comments[a]
Austria	Yes	42.00	26.00	2008	Heavy episodic drinking defined as 60+ g of pure alcohol for men and 40+ g for women at least once during the previous month
Belgium	Yes	26.50	9.90	2009	
Bulgaria	Yes	43.90	23.20	2008	
Cyprus	Yes	48.10	11.90	2009	Heavy episodic drinking defined as six or more glasses of alcoholic beverages on one occasion monthly or more often
Czech Republic	Yes	39.30	19.10	2007	Heavy episodic drinking defined as 80+ g of pure alcohol once a month or more often
Denmark	Yes	38.50	19.20	N/A*	
Estonia	Yes	43.31	12.38	2010	
Finland	Yes	43.00	15.00	2008	Heavy episodic drinking defined as 6+ drinks monthly, which equals 70 g
France	Yes	N/A	N/A	2010	Data not disaggregated by sex; total rate of binge-drinking is 19.00%
Greece	Yes	50.00	33.00	2007	Data from group aged 16 years; heavy episodic drinking defined as 5 or more drinks on one occasion during previous 30 days
Germany	Yes	38.30	13.20	2009	Heavy episodic drinking defined as 5 or more drinks of any alcoholic beverage on a single occasion at least monthly during the previous 12 months (1 heavy episodic drinking occasion was estimated at a minimum of 70 g of ethanol)
Hungary	Yes	17.40	3.70	2007	Heavy episodic drinking defined as getting intoxicated (drunk) from alcohol during the previous 30 days
Ireland	Yes	38.00	17.00	2007	
Italy	Yes	13.40	3.50	2011	Data merged only for >11 years; heavy episodic drinking defined as six or more drinks on one occasion
Latvia	Yes	36.00	20.60	2008	Heavy episodic drinking defined as 60+ g of pure alcohol for males and 40+ g of pure alcohol for females on a single drinking occasion once a month or more often
Lithuania	No	–	–	–	
Luxembourg	Yes	N/A	N/A	2009	
Malta	Yes	N/A	N/A	2008	Heavy episodic drinking defined as at least 48 g of alcohol on one occasion
Netherlands	Yes	44.00	20.00	2009	Heavy episodic drinking defined as six or more glasses of alcohol in one day at least once in the previous six months

Country	National surveys on rates of heavy episodic drinking	Heavy episodic drinking among males (%)	Heavy episodic drinking among females (%)	Year of survey	Comments[a]
Norway	Yes	25.00	10.20	2008	Heavy episodic drinking defined as six or more alcohol units (small bottle of beer, glass of wine) on one occasion more than once per month
Poland	Yes	19.30	2.40	2008	Heavy episodic drinking defined as more than 10 litres of pure 100% alcohol per year for men and 7.5 litres for women
Portugal	Yes	12.20	2.70	2007	Heavy episodic drinking defined as 6+ alcoholic drinks on one drinking occasion, more than once per month, during the previous 12 months
Romania	Yes	N/A	N/A	2009	Heavy episodic drinking defined as five drinks or more on at least one occasion at least once a week; data not disaggregated by sex; total rate of binge-drinking 39.00%
Slovakia	No	–	–	–	
Slovenia	Yes	21.90	4.60	2007	
Spain	Yes	4.80	2.90	2009	
Sweden	Yes	35.30	16.50	N/A	Heavy episodic drinking defined as at least 1 bottle of wine (75 cl) or 5 shot glasses of spirits (25 cl) or 4 cans of beer or cider (>3.5%) or 6 cans of beer (<3.5%), more often than once a week, once a week or 1–3 times per month during the previous 30 days
Switzerland	Yes	15.90	6.30	2007	Heavy episodic drinking defined as 5+ standard drinks (circa 60 g pure alcohol) on one occasion at least every month for men and 4+ standard drinks (circa 48 g of pure alcohol) on one occasion at least every month for women
United Kingdom	Yes	20.40	13.10	2009	Heavy episodic drinking defined as more than eight units for men and six for women on the heaviest drinking day in the previous week

* N/A not available.

[a] Unless otherwise noted, the definition of heavy episodic/binge-drinking is 60+ g of pure alcohol on one occasion, monthly or more often, during the previous 12 months.

Annex 4

CORE FINDINGS AND CONCLUSIONS FOR EU-FINANCED AND CO-FINANCED PROJECTS SINCE 2006

Unrecorded alcohol

Only two of the EC co-financed projects specifically deal with unrecorded alcohol (Gordon & Anderson, 2011). The SMART project is currently developing a survey methodology, which includes unrecorded consumption. While a questionnaire-based methodology appears to be straightforward, some problems regarding unrecorded consumption still exist: people could be buying illegal alcohol without knowing it, and they could refrain from admitting the consumption of unrecorded alcohol due to its illegal status or stigmatization (SMART project, 2012).

The Alcohol Measures for Public Health Research Alliance (AMPHORA) project included a work package that dealt with the chemical analysis and toxicological evaluation of unrecorded alcohol. In a first step of the project, a methodology for sampling, analysis and toxicological evaluation was prepared (Lachenmeier et al., 2011a). In a second step, the methodology was applied to a sample of 115 unrecorded alcohols from 16 European countries. The major findings were that the average alcoholic strength of unrecorded spirits (47.8% volume) was higher compared to recorded spirits. One half of the samples (n=57) showed acceptable alcohol quality. The other half (n=58) showed one or several deficits, with the most prevalent problem being ethyl carbamate contamination (n=29). Other problems included copper (n=20), manganese (n=16) and acetaldehyde (n=12). The magnitude of contamination was, however, judged to be of minor importance for public health as exposure will only in worst-case scenarios reach tolerable daily intakes of these substances. The major problem regarding unrecorded alcohol appeared to be ethanol itself, as it is often higher in strength and its lower price may further contribute to higher drinking amounts. The price of unrecorded alcohol in the AMPHORA sample was approximately 45% of the price of recorded alcohol (Lachenmeier et al., 2011b).

Health sector response

Since 2006, the EC has supported some projects (Gordon & Anderson, 2011) aimed at promoting health sector responses to help reduce alcohol-related problems (Table 4.1).

The Primary Health Care European Project on Alcohol, completed in 2009, aimed to integrate health promotion interventions for hazardous and harmful alcohol consumption into primary care professionals' daily clinical work. The project developed a training programme for primary care professional: clinical guidelines on best practice for health sector purchasers and providers, and a tool to assess the delivery of primary care services for hazardous and harmful drinking.

The AMPHORA project is a four-year (€4 million) initiative with 33 partner organizations from 14 European countries, which started in 2009. AMPHORA aims to pool knowledge and provide new scientific evidence on a range of public health measures to reduce the harm done by alcohol, including on the impact of brief advice and treatment programmes. The project also examines the gap between need for and provision of alcohol interventions in Europe, where the challenges include variations in treatment systems across countries and lack of comparative data on the prevalence of alcohol use disorders.

Table 4.1. EC co-financed and financed projects

Project title and web site	Key activities
Primary Health Care European Project on Alcohol (http://www.phepa.net)	• Development of clinical guidelines and a training manual for brief advice programmes • Development of a tool to assess the delivery of primary care services for hazardous and harmful drinking
AMPHORA (http://amphoraproject.net)	• Production of guidance on evaluating policy interventions • Impact assessment of planned and unplanned social determinants on alcohol consumption • Impact assessment of commercial communications and policy changes in the areas of price and availability • Evaluation of the impact of brief advice and treatment programmes • Documentation of laws and regulations and measuring of the impact of existing alcohol policies • Analysis of public perceptions of drinking problems
Optimizing Delivery of Health Care Interventions (www.odhinproject.eu)	• Identification of evidence to improve acceptance, delivery and maintenance of brief intervention activity in primary care • Modelling studies to test the impact of different brief intervention approaches on changes in alcohol consumption and the resulting impacts on health care costs and health-related quality of life • Randomized controlled trial to evaluate the impact of different promotional strategies on encouraging brief intervention delivery in routine practice • Compilation of an evidence-based database on effective and cost-effective brief intervention measures and a tool to assess the extent of delivery in practice

The Optimizing Delivery of Health Care Interventions project is a four-year study involving nine European countries. The research will help to improve understanding on how best to translate the results of clinical research into everyday practice. The project will use the implementation of brief intervention programmes for hazardous and harmful alcohol consumption in primary health care as a case study. A series of systematic reviews will investigate the impact of different behavioural, organizational and financial strategies in changing providers' behaviour across a range of clinical lifestyle interventions. The knowledge base of potential barriers and facilitators to implementing brief interventions will be updated. A stepped cluster randomized controlled trial will then be undertaken to test the incremental effect of different promotional strategies.

Reducing injuries and death from alcohol-related road crashes

The EU has supported a range of projects focused on alcohol and road safety, with the project Driving under the Influence of Drugs, Alcohol and Medicines (DRUID) among the largest ones (DRUID, 2007). Based on a roadside survey study carried out in 13 countries with almost 50 000 randomly selected drivers, it was concluded that alcohol is still by far the number one psychoactive substance on roads in the EU. Alcohol is estimated to be used by 3.48% of drivers, illicit drugs by 1.9% and medicinal drugs by 1.36%. It was found that "the risk of getting seriously injured or killed when positive for alcohol at 0.5–0.8 g/litre was 2–10 times the risk for sober drivers. The risk increased exponentially: alcohol concentrations of 1.2 g/litre and above increased the risk 20–200 times compared with sober drivers". The risk of being responsible for a crash while driving under the influence of alcohol was found to be three times higher when drugs were also involved. The project also reconfirmed that well-enforced BAC levels below 0.5 g/litre and zero tolerance for young drivers are effective measures in reducing drink–driving.

Drinking environments

Since 2006, the EU has supported a range of projects focusing on reducing harm in drinking environments (Table 4.2). Combined, these have brought together evidence of the effectiveness of interventions, identified examples of practice in European settings, developed tools to increase access to and use of this information, and initiated the process of strengthening the evidence base in European drinking environments.

Table 4.2. EC-financed and co-financed projects since 2006

Project title and web site	Key activities
Focus on Alcohol Safe Environments (FASE) (www.faseproject.eu)	• Conducted a systematic review of evidence from international studies on drinking environments. • Collated case studies from interventions in European drinking environments. • Developed recommendations for policy-makers.
Healthy Nightlife Toolbox (HNT) (www.hnt-info.eu)	Developed an online resource providing access to: • literature and evaluated interventions in drinking environments • experts working in nightlife prevention in European countries • a handbook for practitioners of prevention programmes to help select and implement appropriate preventive interventions.
Alcohol Measures for Public Health Research Alliance (AMPHORA) (www.amphoraproject.net)	Implementing a study in four European drinking environments to: • collect data on nightlife drinking behaviour • identify environmental factors in bars associated with intoxication and alcohol-related harm • provide recommendations for policy-makers.
Club Health (www.club-health.eu)	Developing resources for policy-makers, including: • a database and assessment of nightlife policy • a tool to facilitate local multi-agency partnership working • a set of standards for practice in drinking venues • a training programme for staff working in nightlife settings.
Tourism, Recreation and Violence: A European Level Study (TRAVELS) (www.irefrea.org)	• Conducted a study of substance use, nightlife and harm in European nightlife resorts. • Examined marketing and promotion of risk in holiday resorts • Provided recommendations for policy-makers and tourist organizations.
Ten D by Night (TEND)	• Implemented a study to examine associations between substance use and driving risk in recreational settings. • Tested a preventive intervention to reduce the number and severity of road traffic crashes associated with recreational substance use.

The FASE project reviewed evidence from interventions in drinking environments (Jones, Hughes & Atkinson, 2011) and collected case studies of practice in Europe (Hughes et al., 2010). Recommendations arising from the study included the need: (i) to increase research in Europe to identify the impacts of interventions in drinking environments and improve understanding of nightlife drinking behaviour; (ii) to support local and national bodies in implementing research and accessing its findings; and (iii) to ensure prevention strategies did not focus solely on reducing harm but also on controlling the availability of alcohol and addressing the causes of excessive drinking (Hughes et al., 2010).

The HNT project addressed both alcohol and drug use in drinking environments. It created an online resource for policy-makers and practitioners of prevention programmes to access evidence from interventions in drinking environments, identify and implement appropriate measures and share experience across Europe. The Club Health project is collating and reviewing evidence from nightlife policy in Europe, and developing a range of resources to help local and national partners manage drinking environments. These include: an online resource to facilitate multi-agency partnership working, a set of standards for practice in drinking venues, and a training programme for staff working in nightlife settings.

To strengthen knowledge of alcohol use and harm in drinking environments, the AMPHORA project has conducted a study in four European drinking environments. This has found high levels of alcohol use in young people using bars and nightclubs in all sites, including high levels of preloading and binge-drinking, yet findings have suggested key differences in drinking behaviour between countries.[15] These require further investigation and are likely to be important in understanding the transferability of appropriate preventive interventions. The study will also identify environmental factors in bars associated with intoxication and alcohol-related harm (Hughes et al., 2011b).

The TRAVELS project has focused on substance use, nightlife and violence among European holidaymakers and has identified European holiday resorts as key risk locations for drunkenness and violence (Hughes et al., 2011a) and produced recommendations for policy-makers and tourism organizations (Calafat et al., 2010). To address road traffic crashes associated with substance use in recreational settings, the TEND project has implemented a study in six countries to examine relationships between driving performance and substance use and test a preventive intervention (Siliquini et al., 2010). Findings have yet to be reported.

Alcohol marketing

A range of projects has been funded by the EU to balance the situation where the bulk of research evidence on the impact of alcohol marketing or on the effectiveness of alcohol marketing controls originates outside Europe (Table 4.3).

Original research is ongoing in two projects under the EU Research Framework programme. A longitudinal study within the AMPHORA project is examining the impact of exposure to alcohol-branded sports sponsorship, televised alcohol advertising, digital marketing and alcohol-branded promotional items (The AMPHORA Project, 2010). Research conducted within the Addictions and Lifestyles in Contemporary Europe Reframing Addictions Project (ALICE RAP) is focusing on the effects of exposure to alcohol marketing on brain activity and implicit alcohol expectations among heavy alcohol and cannabis users, as well as the impact of exposure to alcohol marketing on relapse by addicted individuals.

The regulation and self-regulation of alcohol marketing in the EU and, to some extent, across Europe more widely, has been examined in three interlinked projects financed under the EU Health Programme. Project ELSA carried out in 2005–2007 (STAP, 2007a) indicated wide variations in laws, regulations and administrative provisions governing the advertising of alcoholic products. All 24 European countries studied had at least one regulation on the marketing and advertising of alcohol, with a total of 74 regulations. Of these, 45 were at least partly mandated by law and 26 were self-regulatory codes. The collected data show that legislation mainly addresses the volume of alcohol marketing, while self-regulation codes mainly address its content. A Europe-wide literature study found that almost no scientific studies that tested the effectiveness of alcohol marketing regulations in Europe had been published (STAP,

---

[15] Hughes et al. *Drinking behaviours and blood alcohol concentration in four European drinking environments: a cross-sectional study*, unpublished information.

Table 4.3. EU-financed projects on alcohol marketing since 2005

Project title and web site	Key activities	Key findings
Research		
Alcohol Measures for Public Health Research Alliance (AMPHORA) (2009–2012) (www.amphoraproject.net)	A longitudinal study in four European countries on the impact of exposure to alcohol marketing on adolescents' drinking behaviour.	Ongoing
Addictions and Lifestyles in Contemporary Europe Reframing Addictions Project (ALICE RAP) (2011–2015) (http://www.alicerap.eu/)	(i) A neuro-imaging study on the impact of exposure to alcohol marketing on brain activity and implicit association of heavy users. (ii) A longitudinal study of the impact of exposure to alcohol marketing on relapse of alcohol addicts.	Ongoing
Policy		
Enforcement of National Laws and Self-regulation on Advertising and Marketing of Alcohol (ELSA) (2005–2007) (www.elsa-europe.org)	Assessing and reporting on the enforcement of national laws and self-regulation on the advertising and marketing of alcoholic beverages across the EU, applicant countries and Norway.	Statutory regulations mainly address the volume of alcohol marketing. Self-regulation codes mainly address the content of alcohol marketing. Scientific studies to test the effectiveness of alcohol marketing regulations in Europe are rare. There is a lack of an integrated theoretical framework to evaluate the effectiveness of alcohol marketing regulations.
Focus on Alcohol Safe Environments (FASE) (2007–2009) (www.faseproject.eu)	(i) Developing a theoretical framework on the evaluation of alcohol marketing regulations. (ii) Evaluating the effectiveness of alcohol marketing regulations in Europe.	Volume and content restrictions are only effective when there is a strong regulatory system to support enforcement. The regulations in France and Norway are among the best practices in Europe for controlling the volume and content of alcohol advertising.
Alcohol Marketing Monitored in Europe (AMMIE) (2009–2011) (http://www.eucam.info/eucam/home/ammie.html)	(i) Developing a method for monitoring alcohol marketing by public health nongovernmental organizations. (ii) Monitoring alcohol marketing in five EU countries. (iii) Testing the effectiveness of alcohol marketing legislation and self-regulation in five EU countries.	Existing alcohol marketing regulations and, more specifically, self-regulation codes are ineffective in protecting young people against exposure to large numbers of alcohol marketing practices.

2007b). More importantly, no integrated theoretical framework to evaluate the effectiveness of existing alcohol marketing regulations was found. The FASE project carried out in 2007–2009 set out to fill this gap by developing a framework for evaluating alcohol marketing policy interventions (de Bruijn, Johansen & van den Broeck 2010). The framework was used to evaluate existing alcohol marketing regulations across Europe (de Bruijn, 2011). It was concluded that restrictions on volume and content are only effective when a strong regulatory system supports their enforcement. Alcohol marketing regulations in France and Norway were considered among the best practices in Europe, with strict volume or content restrictions accompanied by a strong supportive regulatory system.

The Alcohol Marketing Monitored in Europe (AMMIE) project extended knowledge about the effectiveness of existing alcohol marketing regulations in Europe by monitoring alcohol marketing in five European countries. The monitoring method was developed and carried out systematically by public health nongovernmental organizations. The results indicate that existing alcohol marketing regulations and self-regulatory codes are ineffective in protecting young people against exposure to large volumes of alcohol marketing.

Effectiveness and cost–effectiveness

The Eurocare project, Alcohol Policy Network in the Context of a Larger Europe: Bridging the Gap (Eurocare, 2012), scaled alcohol policies across 28 countries in 2005 ranging from 0 (no policy) to 40 (maximum policy).The scales ranged from 4 to 35.5, with a mean of 13.5. While there was no relationship between score on the scale and per capita alcohol consumption in the group aged 15+ years in countries with a score less than the mean (regression standardized beta = -0.28, p = 0.39), there was a significant relationship between score on the scale and per capita alcohol consumption in that group for countries with a score more than the mean: the higher the score, the lower the alcohol consumption (regression standardized beta = -0.57, p = 0.04).

Analysis of 15 EU countries from the ECAS project for 1970–2000, which used a 20-point scale, found that the mean score increased from 8.7 in 1970 to 11.4 in 1990, remaining 11.4 in 2000. Over the 30-year period, there was a highly significant relationship between the ECAS score and per capita alcohol consumption: the higher the score, the lower the alcohol consumption (regression standardized beta = -0.68, p = less than 0.000) (Fig. 4.1). The relationship between a higher score and lower alcohol consumption increased from 1970 to 1990 and then declined in 2000. While there were relationships between the ECAS score and deaths from liver cirrhosis and between the ECAS score and deaths from a range of alcohol-related conditions (increased score, lower death rates), the relationship was fully explained by the relationship between the ECAS score and per capita alcohol consumption.

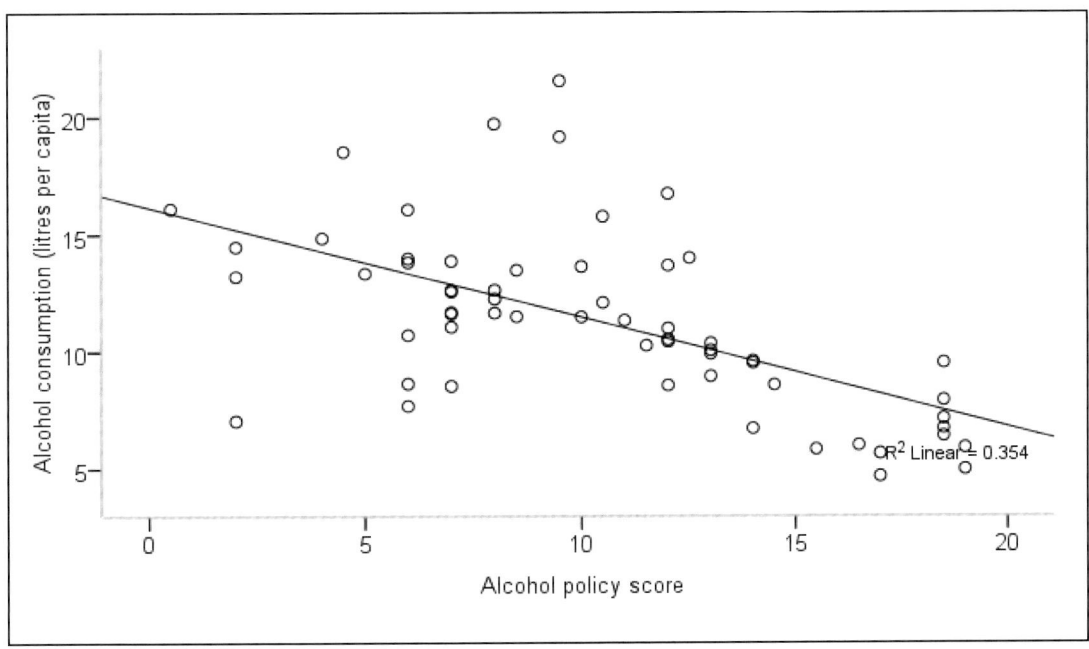

Fig. 4.1. Scatterplot between ECAS policy score and per capita alcohol consumption, 15 EU countries for the 4 years 1970, 1980, 1990, 2000

The Building Capacity project undertook a health and economic impact assessment of a range of alcohol policies in 22 European countries (Chisholm et al., 2009). The assessment demonstrates that country contextualization can change the cost–effectiveness ratios. For example, compared with the other Eur-C countries, costs per DALY averted in Estonia were cheaper for taxation, an advertising ban and roadside breath-testing, and more expensive for reduced access and brief advice in primary care. Thus, in Estonia, in contrast to the rest of the Eur-C countries, an advertising ban became more cost–effective than reduced access, and roadside breath-testing became more cost–effective than brief advice in primary care.

The SMART project considered the costs and benefits of alcohol policy using, as an example, a hypothetical tax increase on alcohol that would result in an across the board 10% price increase in England (Anderson & Baumberg, 2010), based on data derived from the Sheffield alcohol policy model (Purshouse et al., 2009).

The analysis concluded that, at an implementation cost of €3.7 million, a tax increase would bring benefits worth €588 million – a figure that would be even higher if the benefits accruing to people other than drinkers were included. This favourable balance would need to be adjusted, once accurate estimates of the probably rather small transition costs to the alcohol industry were added (although such costs could be covered from extra government tax revenue). The value of the non-tangible costs and benefits estimated that the benefits in terms of the value of improved quality of life (€110 million) outweighed the estimated value that consumers might have placed on their lost drinks (€54 million).

References

AMPHORA. The AMPHORA project [web site] (2010). Brussels, European Commission (http://amphora project.net, accessed 13 February 2012).

Anderson P, Baumberg B (2010). *Cost benefit analyses of alcohol policy – a primer*. Warsaw, Institute of Psychiatry and Neurology.

Calafat A et al. (2010). *Tourism, nightlife and violence: a cross cultural analysis and preventive recommendations*. Palma de Mallorca, IREFREA.

Chisholm D et al. (2009). *Alcohol policy cost–effectiveness briefing notes for 22 European countries*. London, Institute of Alcohol Studies.

de Bruijn A (2011). *Alcohol marketing regulations in Europe: how effective are they?* Utrecht, European Centre for Monitoring Alcohol Marketing (EUCAM fact sheet).

de Bruijn A, Johansen I, van den Broeck A (2010). *Effective alcohol marketing regulations: a proposed framework to evaluate existing alcohol marketing regulations*. Utrecht, Dutch Institute for Alcohol Policy.

DRUID – Driving under the Influence of Drugs, Alcohol and Medicines [web site] (2007). Bergisch Gladbach-Bensberg, Federal Highway Research Institute (http://www.druid-project.eu/cln_031/nn_107548/Druid/EN/about-DRUID/about-DRUID-node.html?__nnn=true, accessed 12 February 2012).

Eurocare (2012). Alcohol Policy Network in the Context of a Larger Europe: Bridging the Gap [web site]. Brussels, European Commission (http://www.ias.org.uk/btg/index.html, accessed 24 February 2012).

Gordon R, Anderson P (2011). Science and alcohol policy: a case study of EU strategy on alcohol. *Addiction*, 106(S1):55–66.

Hughes K et al. (2010). *Reducing harm in drinking environments: policy briefing*. Liverpool, Centre for Public Health, Liverpool John Moores University.

Hughes K et al. (2011a). Substance use, violence, and unintentional injury in young holidaymakers visiting Mediterranean destinations. *Journal of Travel Medicine,* 18(2):80–89.

Hughes K et al. (2011b). Environmental factors in drinking venues and alcohol-related harm: the evidence base for European intervention. *Addiction,* 106(S1):37–46.

Jones L, Hughes K, Atkinson AM (2011). Reducing harm in drinking environments: a systematic review of effective approaches. *Health & Place*, 17(2):508–518.

Lachenmeier DW et al. (2011a). Is contaminated alcohol a health problem in the European Union? A review of existing and methodological outline for future studies. *Addiction*, 106(Suppl.1):20–30.

Lachenmeier DW et al. (2011b) Quality of illegally and informally produced alcohol in Europe: results from the AMPHORA project. *Adicciones*, 23:133–140.

Purshouse R et al. (2009). *Modelling to assess the effectiveness and cost–effectiveness of public health related strategies and interventions to reduce alcohol attributable harm in England using the Sheffield Alcohol Policy Model version 2.0. Report to the NICE Public Health Programme Development Group.* Sheffield, University of Sheffield, School of Health and Related Research (ScHARR).

Siliquini R et al. (2010). A European study on alcohol and drug use among young drivers: the TEND by Night study design and methodology. *BMC Public Health,* 10:205.

SMART project. Minutes of the European Conference on Standardizing Measurement of Alcohol Troubles (SMART). Barcelona, 19 October 2010 [web site]. Warsaw, Institute of Psychiatry and Neurology, 2012 (http://www.ipin.edu.pl/alcsmart/meetings_and_conference_01.html, accessed 17 February 2012).

STAP (2007a). *Regulation of alcohol marketing in Europe. Vol. 2.* Utrecht, National Institute for Alcohol Policy (STAP).

STAP (2007b). *Report on adherence to alcohol marketing regulations. Vol. 3.* Utrecht, National Institute for Alcohol Policy (STAP).

The WHO Regional Office for Europe

The World Health Organization (WHO) is a specialized agency of the United Nations created in 1948 with the primary responsibility for international health matters and public health. The WHO Regional Office for Europe is one of six regional offices throughout the world, each with its own programme geared to the particular health conditions of the countries it serves.

Member States

Albania
Andorra
Armenia
Austria
Azerbaijan
Belarus
Belgium
Bosnia and Herzegovina
Bulgaria
Croatia
Cyprus
Czech Republic
Denmark
Estonia
Finland
France
Georgia
Germany
Greece
Hungary
Iceland
Ireland
Israel
Italy
Kazakhstan
Kyrgyzstan
Latvia
Lithuania
Luxembourg
Malta
Monaco
Montenegro
Netherlands
Norway
Poland
Portugal
Republic of Moldova
Romania
Russian Federation
San Marino
Serbia
Slovakia
Slovenia
Spain
Sweden
Switzerland
Tajikistan
The former Yugoslav
   Republic of Macedonia
Turkey
Turkmenistan
Ukraine
United Kingdom
Uzbekistan

Alcohol in the European Union
Consumption, harm and policy approaches

World Health Organization Regional Office for Europe
Scherfigsvej 8, DK-2100 Copenhagen Ø, Denmark
Tel.: +45 39 17 17 17. Fax: +45 39 17 18 18. E-mail: contact@euro.who.int
Web site: www.euro.who.int